IMAGES
of America

MONTANA'S
HOT SPRINGS

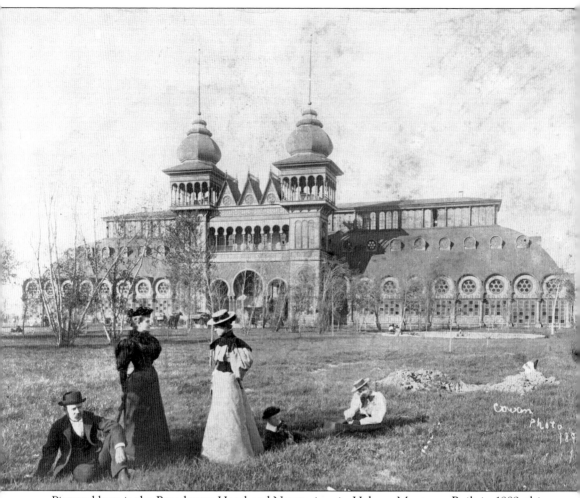

Pictured here is the Broadwater Hotel and Natatorium in Helena, Montana. Built in 1889, this elegant resort was one of the most extravagant hot springs developments in the United States. The hot-water pool in the natatorium was as big as a football field. A cascade of hot and cold waterfalls plunged from a 40-foot-tall granite outcropping into the giant pool. (Author's collection.)

ON THE COVER: These bathers are pictured in 1890 at Lolo Hot Springs near the Idaho/Montana border. First visited by explorers Meriwether Lewis and William Clark in 1805, Lolo Hot Springs became a popular recreation spot for Missoula residents. (Author's collection.)

IMAGES
of America

MONTANA'S
HOT SPRINGS

Jeff Birkby

ARCADIA
PUBLISHING

Published by Arcadia Publishing
Charleston, South Carolina

Printed in the United States of America

Library of Congress Control Number: 2017958426

For all general information, please contact Arcadia Publishing:
Telephone 843-853-2070
Fax 843-853-0044
E-mail sales@arcadiapublishing.com
For customer service and orders:
Toll-Free 1-888-313-2665

Visit us on the Internet at www.arcadiapublishing.com

*Dedicated to the men and women who had
the vision to develop simple springs of hot water into
Montana's first social and recreational centers*

CONTENTS

ACKNOWLEDGMENTS

My sincere thanks go to all Montana hot springs owners who have shared their stories and personal memorabilia. Thanks also to the staff of many county and state historical societies in Montana for their enthusiastic assistance with finding old hot springs photographs in their archives. Also, a thank you goes to Stacia Bannerman of Arcadia Publishing for her patience and guidance over the course of completing this book.

Images in this volume appear courtesy of the Montana Historical Society Research Center Photograph Archives (MHS), the University of Montana Archives (UM), the Historical Museum at Fort Missoula (HMFM), the Montana State University Archives (MSU), the Ravalli County Museum (RCM), the Beaverhead County Museum (BCM), the Larue–Hot Springs Museum (HSM), and the Yellowstone Gateway Museum of Park County (YGM).

All uncredited photographs are from the author's personal collection.

INTRODUCTION

The 19th century was a period of discovery in Montana. Among the natural features that impressed new visitors to the area were Montana's myriad hot springs, which steamed and bubbled on valley floors, by powerful rivers, and on the open prairies. As increasing numbers of settlers and gold miners arrived in Montana after the end of the Civil War, word spread of these mysterious pockets of artesian hot water that poured out of the earth.

Many of the pioneers who traveled to Montana in the 1860s and 1870s were European immigrants with memories of family and locations in Germany, Austria, and other Central European countries. These countries had rich histories of using hot springs for health and recreation, and the tradition of "taking the waters" for relaxation and therapy was well known. When these immigrants arrived in Montana, some of them realized the potential of commercializing these untamed geothermal resources into bathing resorts similar to those they had known in Europe.

These new immigrants also saw that Native American tribes in Montana already had discovered and valued Montana's hot springs. Dr. A.J. Hunter, arriving by wagon train to Montana in 1864, stopped near some hot springs on the Yellowstone River. Dr. Hunter observed more than 1,000 members of the Crow Indian tribe encamped near the thermal waters, where they were bathing their sick and elderly tribal members.

By the early 1880s, many of Montana's hot springs had been "claimed" by new immigrants who filed homestead claims on the land. The natural flows of thermal water were diverted into crude log soaking pools, which were sometimes covered with a log cabin. These hot springs were often the only place where a dusty miner or tired rancher could get a hot bath.

As the years progressed, many of these simple soaking pools were enlarged into more civilized recreation centers with dressing rooms, restaurants, and simple hotels built nearby for the bathers. The larger developments became social centers where picnics and dances were held.

An 1880s newspaper article describing the thermal waters near the Montana town of Deer Lodge captured the appeal of Montana's frontier hot springs: "The business man whose vital powers are impaired by constant labor at his desk, the overworked mechanic whose tired body calls for rest, the care-worn wife whose manifold household duties have overtaxed her weak form, the literary man whose wearied brain demands relaxation from toil, the day laborer who wants a holiday, and all others suffering from the ills to which flesh is heir can find no better place to recuperate and regain lost health and strength than at the deservedly popular Warm Springs of the Deer Lodge Valley."

A handful of Montana hot springs resorts grew into vacation oases that rivaled the elegant spas of Europe. Hunter's Hot Springs, Corwin Hot Springs, Broadwater Hot Springs, and Boulder Hot Springs were among the Montana resorts that flourished in the 1900s. But most of Montana's sumptuous resorts faded from time and memory as the dream of large urban populations arriving to support these grand developments never materialized.

Montana's hot springs may never again see an era of elegance as they did in the early 20th century. However, the images captured in photographs and postcards from that time will help future generations remember that Montana's hot springs resorts offered respite and culture for all—gold and copper miners, ranchers, shopkeepers, and politicians alike.

On January 7, 1886, this poem by an unknown author appeared in the *Rocky Mountain Husbandman*. The poem captured the fascination and appeal of the hot springs on Montana's frontier:

Oh! Fountain of perpetual youth,
we hail with joy the evincing truth:
that in thy magic water is rife,
a balm for all the ills of life.

And nowhere in this world is found,
save on this very hallowed ground—
of pharmacist's or Nature's compound—
a remedy, in which there doth abound
a healing power that can compare
with thy boiling fluid, pure and fair.

In thee is beauty for the faded cheek.
an appetizer for the faint and weak;
the lame to leap and the blind to see,
the old rheumatic from pain set free.

Dyspeptic's life in thee is saved,
old age snatched from verge of the grave;
eternal youth and beauty divine,
to the sons and daughters of every clime,
who, in thy crystal pools do dip,
or from this sparkling fountain sip.

One

SIMPLE RUSTIC
MONTANA SOAKS

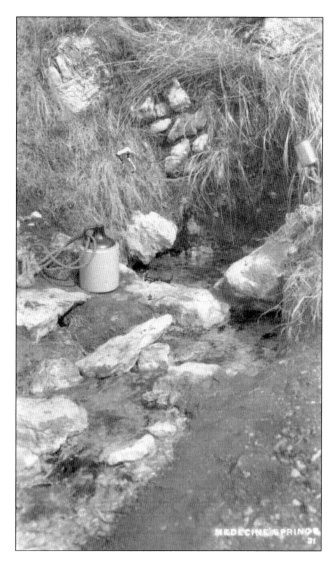

All of Montana's developed hot springs were at one time simple pools of hot water where pioneers would submerge their aching bodies for a relaxing soak. Many of these remained open bathing pools with rough timbers cut to surround the pool or, at most, a crude log cabin covering the spring to protect bathers from harsh winter winds. Some were a bit further developed, perhaps supporting a more civilized bathhouse with a dressing room. These smaller rural pools either faded with time or remained simple soaking venues that retain their charm. Examples of these smaller thermal Montana soaks include Sun River Hot Springs, Norris Hot Springs, Byrne Resort, Camp Aqua, and Montaqua. This image shows a drinking jug next to Sun River Hot Springs.

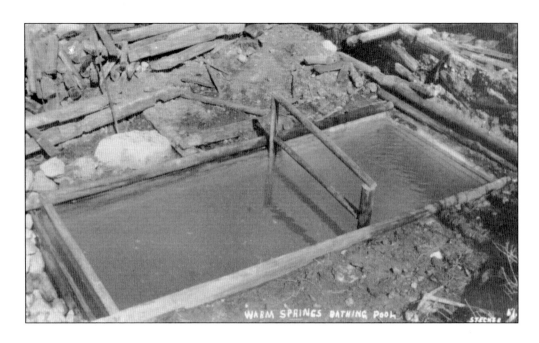

Sun River Hot Springs are located 60 miles west of Great Falls. The rustic springs were also called Alta Mineral Springs, Lockey's Mineral Springs, and Medicine Springs. By 1886, a crude bathhouse had been constructed over the springs. Visitors included the painter Charlie Russell, who traveled to the springs from his home in Great Falls in 1898. A mineral-rich deposit of clay salts near the springs gained fame for their curative properties. A company in New York City marketed the clay salts as "Sun River Ointment" that could cure many skin ailments. The hot springs were developed by a guest ranch in the late 1920s and purchased by the K Bar L Ranch in 1947. (Both, MHS.)

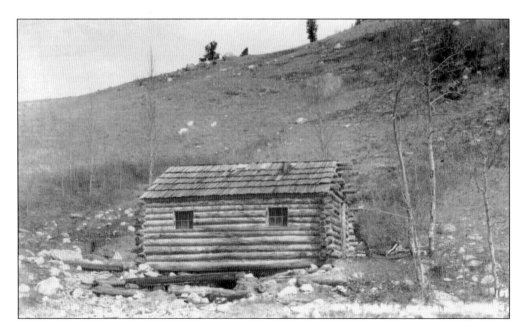

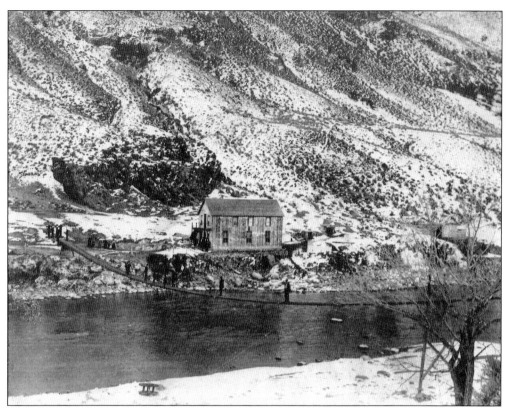

Julius LaDuke, a French-Canadian immigrant, built the LaDuke Hot Springs Resort in 1899. The hot springs were located just a few miles north of Yellowstone National Park on the banks of the Yellowstone River. The simple bathhouse contained a plunge bath as well as wooden tubs. LaDuke built a small two-story hotel next to the plunge. The resort attracted Yellowstone-bound visitors who would stay for a night or two before entering the park. A 1902 article in the *Wonderland Newspaper* stated that the hot springs were "equal of any springs in the west, and are a positive cure for all diseases that hot springs are calculated to cure." In 1905, a similar article added that the "springs enjoy an enviable reputation for the relief of rheumatism, gout, neuralgia, sciatica and disorders of the heart, kidneys, stomach, and nervous system." (Both, YGM.)

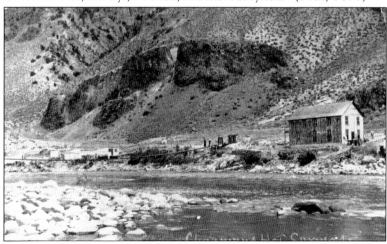

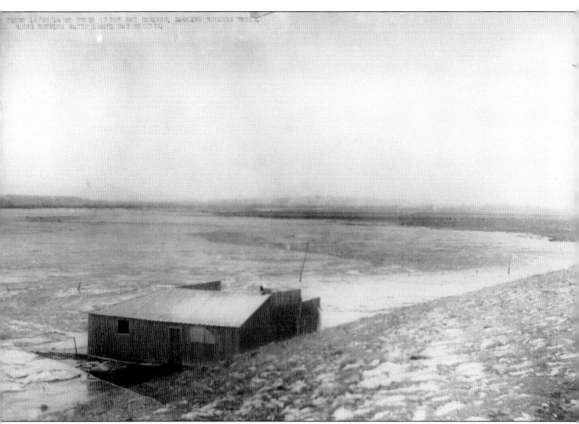

This photograph of the Thexton Hot Springs bathhouse was taken in December 1914. Thexton Hot Springs are located two miles north of the town of Ennis in southwest Montana and surrounded by the Madison, Tobacco Root, and Gravelly Mountain Ranges. The springs issued from the west bank of a terrace above the Madison River. Thexton Hot Springs were developed for public bathing and swimming in the 1880s. With surface temperatures above 180 degrees Fahrenheit, these springs have what is likely the hottest temperature of any hot springs in Montana.

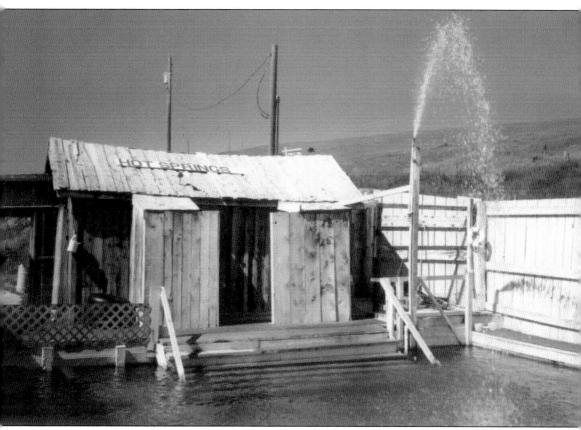

Norris Hot Springs, an open-air pool about 30 miles west of Bozeman, was homesteaded by Charles Hapgood in the 1860s. A wagon train captain on the Bozeman Trail commented that the "water was so hot that if you put your hand in it, you would jerk it out quick without anyone telling you to. It is the devil's teapot, and Hell could not be far off." The hot water was channeled into a pipe that shot the water about 15 feet in the air. The shower of hot water cooled to a pleasant bathing temperature as it fell into the soaking pool. The 30-by-40-foot pool was about four feet deep, with a wooden bench lining the sides. The hot springs had several owners through the decades, including a local community club that managed the hot springs in the 1930s.

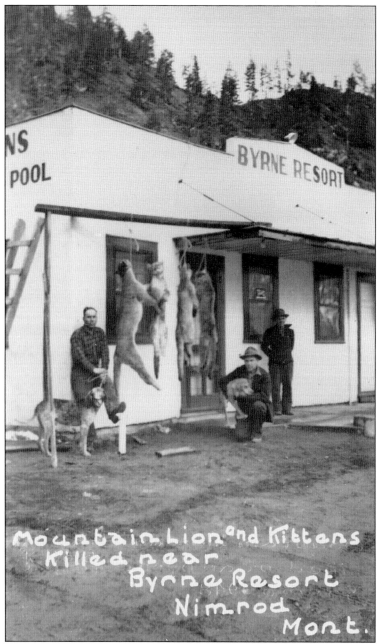

Mountain Lion and Kittens Killed near Byrne Resort Nimrod Mont.

L.P. Byrne, an engineer for the Northern Pacific Railway, built a small resort at Nimrod Warm Springs about 30 miles east of Missoula. The springs cascaded from a rock cliff into a pool that flowed into the Clark Fork River. In 1930, Byrne built a 25-by-60-foot swimming pool blasted out of solid rock next to the springs. He also built a small store, gas station, and restaurant next to the swimming pool, and he named the development Byrne Resort. The resort was a popular stop for travelers going between Butte and Missoula. The water temperature in the springs rarely exceeded 70 degrees, so the swimming pool was most popular in the warmer summer months. Hunters also frequented the resort, which had easy access to the Garnet Mountains. Byrne died in January 1945. No traces of the resort remain today. (MHS.)

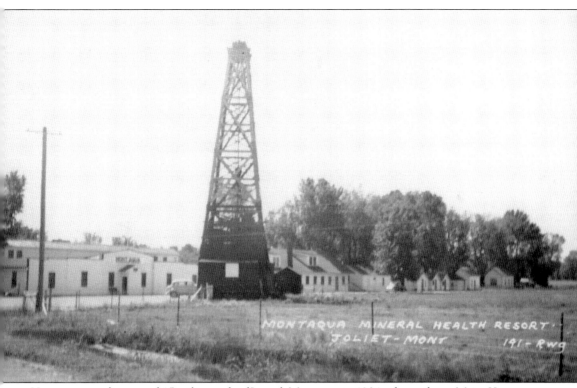

Hot water was discovered 15 miles south of Laurel, Montana, in 1904, when oilman Major Keown drilled 4,000 feet down into a 112-degrees-Fahrenheit aquifer. Keown built the Montaqua Mineral Health Resort around the hot-water well. The small resort featured a bathhouse, a restaurant, and tourist cabins. The resort came to a sudden end on August 17, 1959, when the hot water abruptly stopped flowing from the well. The cause of the sudden loss of water was an earthquake east of Yellowstone National Park and about 100 miles west of Montaqua. The quake registered at 7.3 on the Richter scale—perhaps the strongest earthquake ever recorded in Montana. The underground geology was apparently disturbed by the distant earthquake. The resort could not afford to drill a new well and permanently closed. (MHS.)

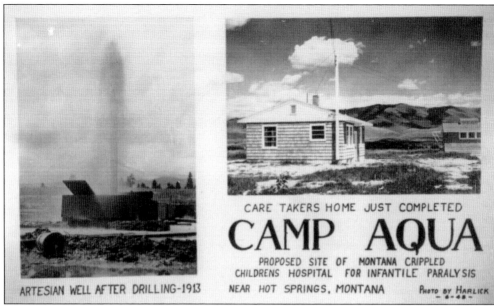

ARTESIAN WELL AFTER DRILLING-1913

CARE TAKERS HOME JUST COMPLETED

CAMP AQUA

PROPOSED SITE OF MONTANA CRIPPLED
CHILDRENS HOSPITAL FOR INFANTILE PARALYSIS

NEAR HOT SPRINGS, MONTANA

Photo by Harlick
- 6-48 -

Mollie Bartlett homesteaded land seven miles east of the town of Hot Springs, Montana. Seeking a source of water for her parched garden, Bartlett drilled a well in 1912 that produced hot water with so much force that the drillers were drenched. Bartlett's small homestead house was located near the gushing well, and the forceful stream of water threatened to undercut the home's foundation. Teams of horses were hooked to the home, and it was dragged a few yards away from the encroaching water. In 1941, Bartlett developed the well into a small resort that she called Camp Aqua, then started a campaign called "Montana's Warm Water Project for Crippled Children." The project brought Montana children suffering from polio to the small resort for therapeutic treatments in the hot water.

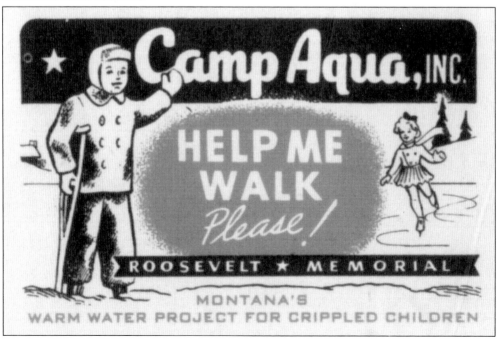

Camp Aqua, INC.

HELP ME
WALK
Please!

ROOSEVELT ★ MEMORIAL

MONTANA'S
WARM WATER PROJECT FOR CRIPPLED CHILDREN

Two

MEDIUM-SIZED
MONTANA RESORTS

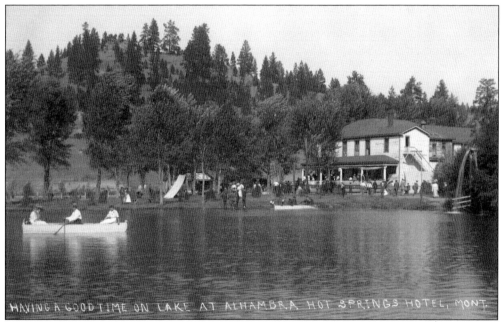

HAVING A GOOD TIME ON LAKE AT ALHAMBRA HOT SPRINGS HOTEL, MONT.

As Montana's population grew in the late 19th century, some of its hot springs were developed into larger and more civilized resorts. Rustic soaking pools were piped into larger plunges and swimming pools, hotels containing dining rooms and dance halls were added, and train service and stagecoach connections brought larger crowds to these more developed resorts. Hot springs often became social centers for the surrounding community, as locals would gather for birthday celebrations, company parties, reunions, and wedding celebrations. Several of these developments also garnered reputations as health and wellness centers. Examples of these medium-sized resorts include Gregson Hot Springs, Alhambra Hot Springs, White Sulphur Springs, and the Symes Hotel. Alhambra Hot Springs is pictured above. (MHS.)

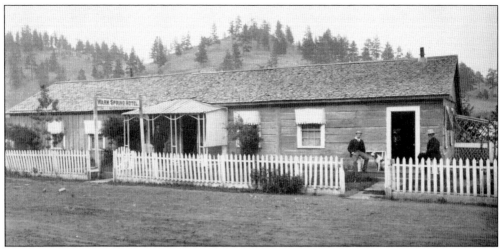

Sylvenius Dustin homesteaded Alhambra Hot Springs south of Helena in the early 1860s. In 1866, Dustin was approached by Wilson Redding, who purchased the land and hot springs from Dustin for $3,000 in gold dust. Redding built the first log hotel at the hot springs that same year. Since the hotel was located so close to the developing gold-rush town of Helena, gold miners were frequent visitors to the little resort.

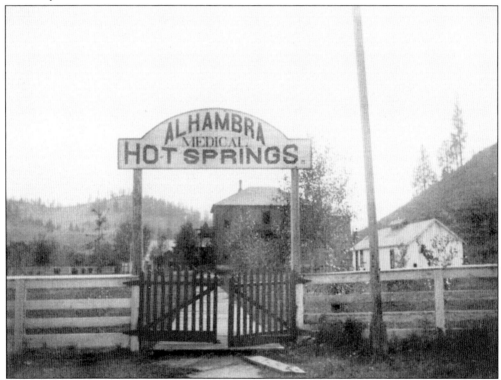

The medicinal properties of the hot springs at Alhambra were promoted as a cure-all. *Northwest Magazine* reported in 1891 that "workers in the mines and smelters of Montana have found the waters in some of the springs to contain the proper antidote against lead, arsenic, and zinc poisoning, and even the worst stages of rheumatism and gout have been successfully treated where other remedies have repeatedly failed."

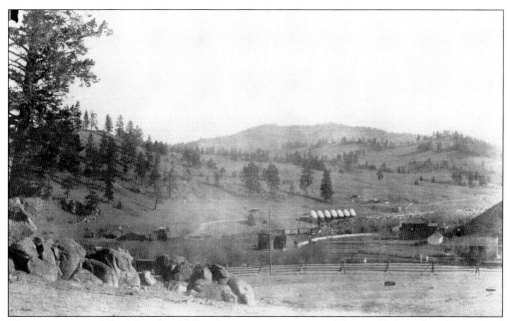

These two views of the Alhambra Valley show a prominent row of charcoal kilns. The whitewashed kilns were used to produce high-quality charcoal by burning wood with little oxygen present. Charcoal produced a much hotter fire than wood when it was burned, which made the charcoal valuable for use in the smelting of gold ore. (Both, MHS.)

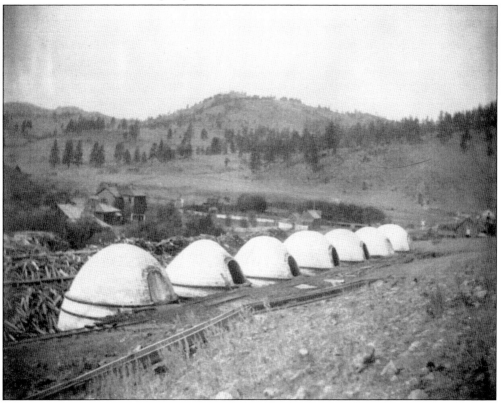

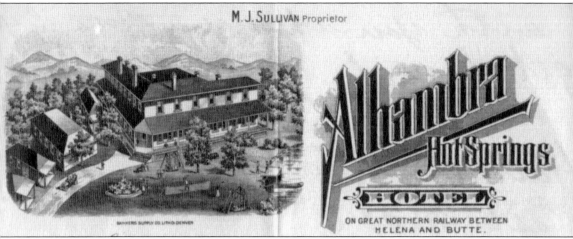

M.J. Sullivan expanded the facilities at Alhambra Hot Springs after he purchased the property in 1904. His 65-room hotel featured steam heat and electric lights. Bathing facilities were available within the hotel, including vapor baths, mud baths, and hot-water plunge baths. Sullivan also built a large swimming pool adjacent to the hotel.

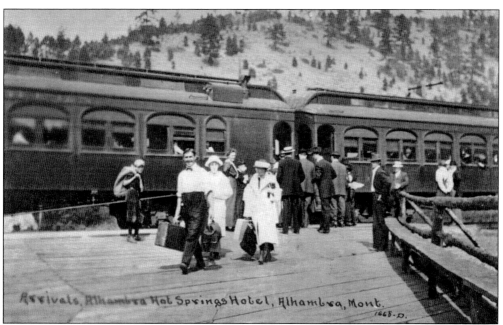

Arrivals, Alhambra Hot Springs Hotel, Alhambra, Mont. 1668-D.

The Great Northern Railway built a rail stop at Alhambra in 1888, which proved to be a boon for the resort. By the early 1920s, at least eight daily trains dropped off passengers at Alhambra. The trains also carried a tank car filled with Alhambra mineral water to Great Falls, where it was bottled and sold commercially. The mineral water was also available at several drinking fountains on the hotel grounds. Unfortunately, the mineral water was found to be radioactive and therefore unfit to drink. (Both, MHS.)

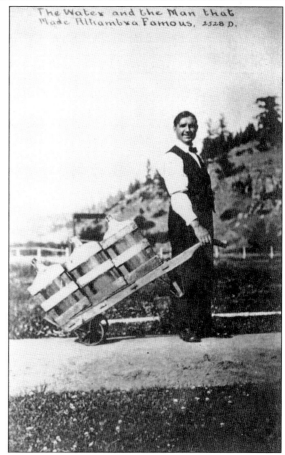

The Water and the Man that Made Alhambra Famous. 2528 D.

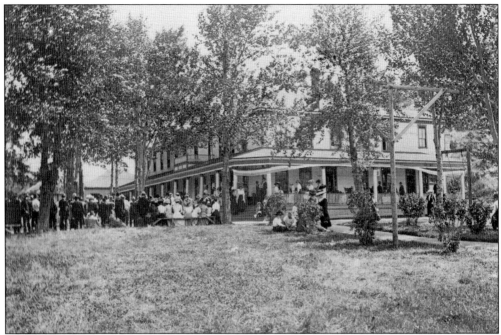

The Alhambra Hot Springs Hotel, an elegant white-framed building with green shutters, a spacious lawn, and large shade trees, was the site of many social events for Helena visitors. The hotel's restaurant featured "incomparable chicken dinners." Guests paid about $20 per week for room, board, and hot springs soaks. The hotel was destroyed in a spectacular fire on April 24, 1959; the *Great Falls Tribune* reported that only items saved from the flames were "a piano and a little beer."

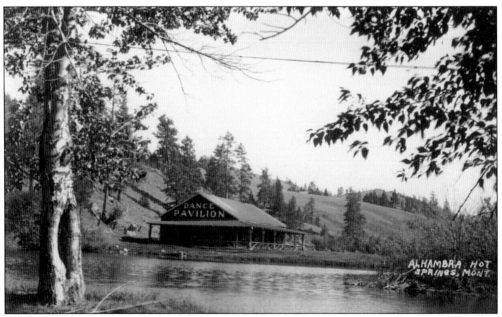

A dance pavilion and lake provided visitors with recreational and social opportunities while visiting the Alhambra resort.

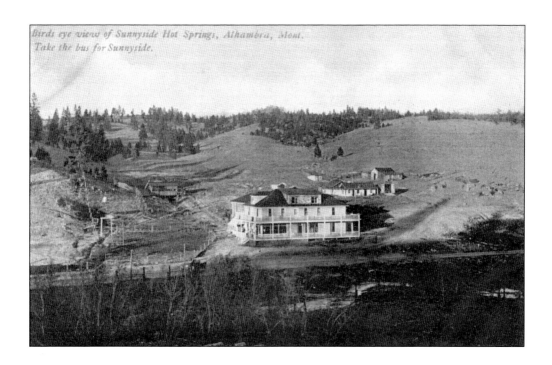

Birds eye view of Sunnyside Hot Springs, Alhambra, Mont.
Take the bus for Sunnyside.

The hot springs resource at Alhambra was shared by two hotels—Alhambra Hot Springs Resort and Sunnyside Hotel. Both hotels were in operation until the 1950s. Sunnyside was the site of many state conventions, including the annual meeting of the Montana Master Plumber's Association in 1910.

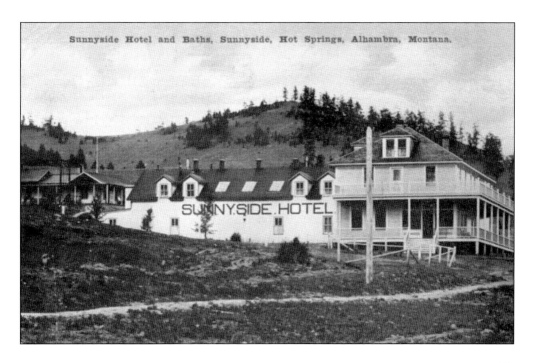

Sunnyside Hotel and Baths, Sunnyside, Hot Springs, Alhambra, Montana.

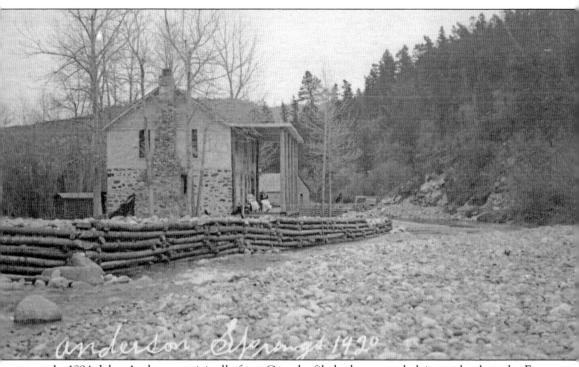

Anderson Springs 1920

In 1894, John Anderson, originally from Canada, filed a homestead claim on land on the East Boulder River about 35 miles south of Big Timber. A warm spring containing lithia gas was located on the property, and Anderson built a hotel, bathhouse, and swimming pool to take advantage of it. Anderson directed the flow of the 70-degree spring into a swimming pool and bathhouse. The spring's rate of flow varied with the seasons, reaching a high of 45 gallons per minute in midsummer but producing significantly less in the winter months. The springs gained a reputation for being able to cure arthritis and other ailments via drinking and bathing in the warm lithia water. In addition to the hotel and pool, Anderson added tents and cabins to the land, which became a popular gathering spot in warmer months. Anderson died on October 12, 1915, and the ownership of the springs changed hands several times after his death. (YGM.)

A Bozeman wagon-maker named Jeremiah Mathews discovered hot springs west of Bozeman in 1879. Mathews built a bathhouse and plunge bath at the site, which he called Mathews' Warm Springs. E. Myron Ferris (pictured) purchased the springs from Mathews in 1890 for $25,000. Ferris changed the name of the plunge to Ferris Hot Springs and built a two-story hotel, a second plunge, and private baths. (MSU.)

Ferris Hot Springs were located eight miles west of Bozeman, and Ferris provided transportation from the city to any potential guests who wanted to visit the springs. Ferris built this horse-drawn herdic, a fancy coach with open sides, and used it to bring guests to the resort. (MSU.)

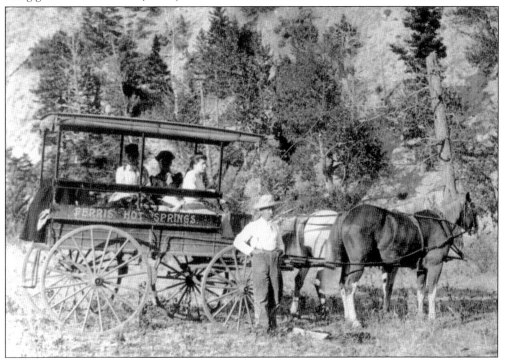

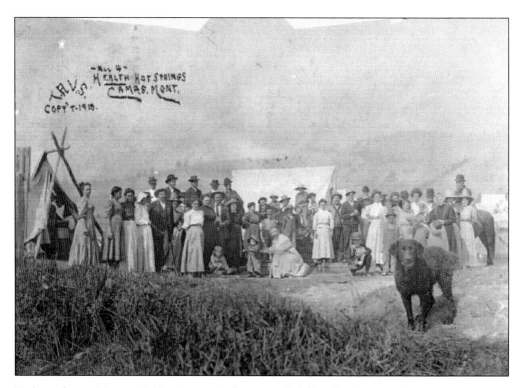

Early settlers in Montana's Hot Springs Valley west of Flathead Lake enjoyed soaking in the hot, mineral-rich mud at Camas Hot Springs. The first soaking pool at Camas Hot Springs was built by Ed Lemoreux around 1905. The eight-foot-square open-air pool was used until 1911. Soaking was free to the public. A local newspaper, the *Sanders County Signal*, encouraged visitors to soak in and drink the water to relieve "the grumps," which the newspaper stated was a condition that "makes one find fault with his surroundings."

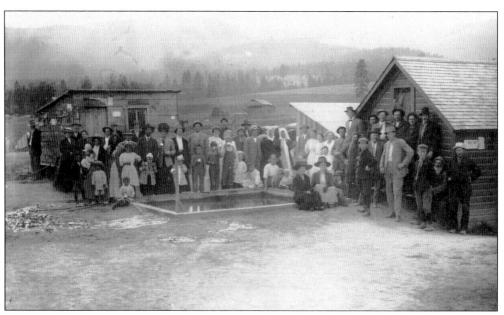

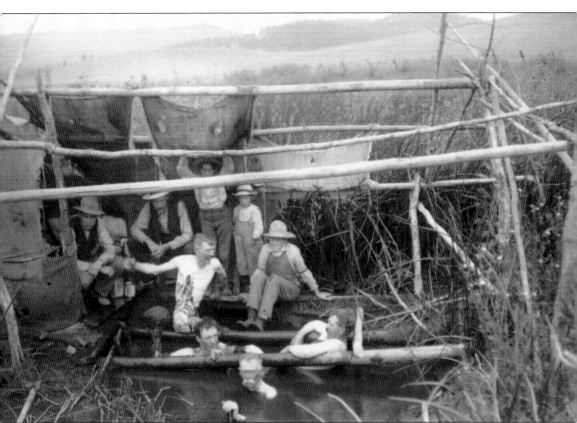

One of the few natural hot mud baths in Montana, the open-air bath at Camas was a popular venue for treating skin diseases as well as providing a relaxing break to farmers and ranchers in the Hot Springs Valley.

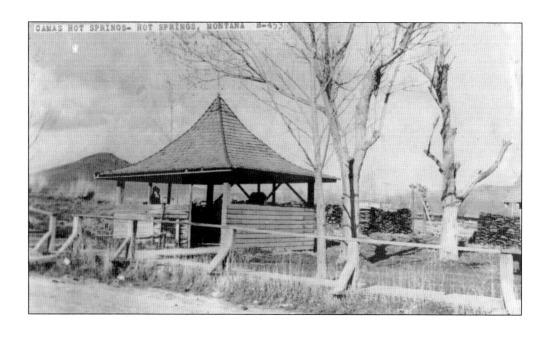

Here are two views of the Fountain of Youth gazebo that covered one of the hot springs at Camas. Many cures were ascribed to the power of the hot water and mud at Camas Hot Springs. The *Camas Hot Springs Exchange* reported that "a gentleman came here who had no hair on the top of his head. He daily bathed and massaged his scalp with the hot springs water and left here with a new growth covering the once sensitive spot. This is encouraging."

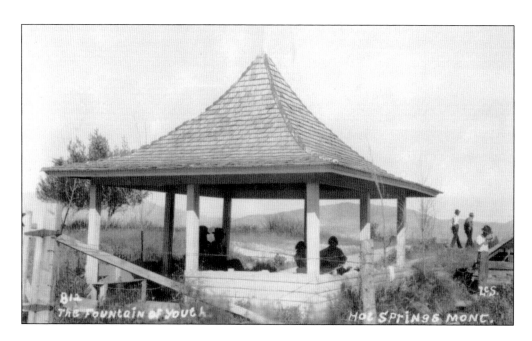

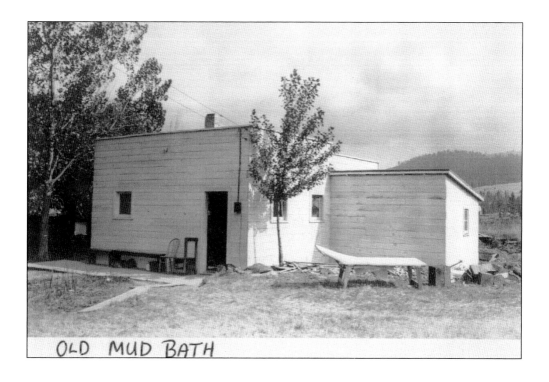

OLD MUD BATH

The first enclosed bathhouse at Camas Hot Springs was built in 1911. This enclosure contained seven rooms and eight bathtubs.

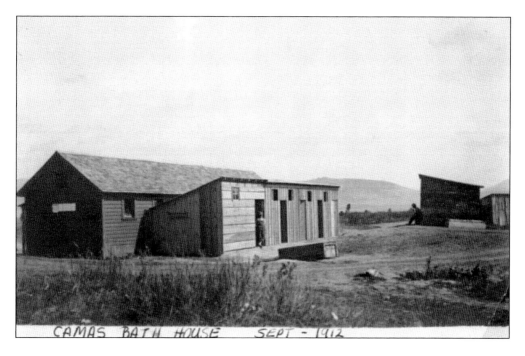

CAMAS BATH HOUSE   SEPT - 1912

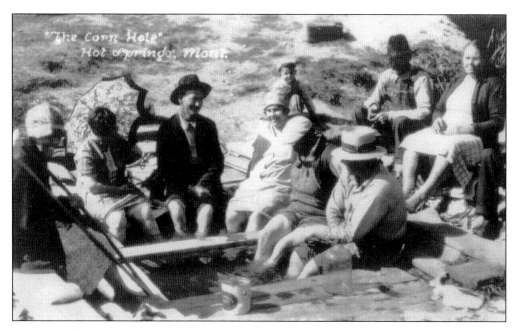

A unique thermal feature found at no other hot springs resort in Montana is the Camas "corn hole," a shallow pit of naturally bubbling hot mud that was surrounded with flat boards. Visitors would sit on the edge of the pit and dangle their feet and lower legs in the mud. The treatment was thought to be especially effective in treating corns and bunions on the feet, which is how the mud bath acquired the nickname "corn hole." The above photograph shows the corn hole in 1911. (Note that one of the women has a crutch; perhaps she was soaking in the hot water to help with arthritis in her leg.) The below image is of women soaking their feet in the corn hole around 1940.

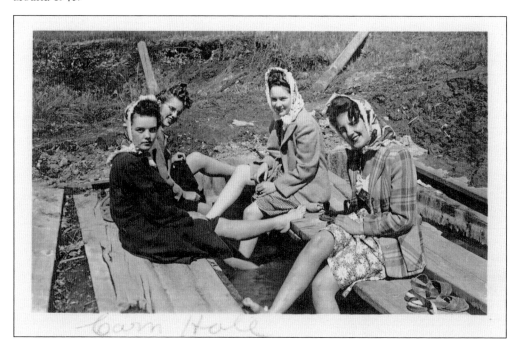

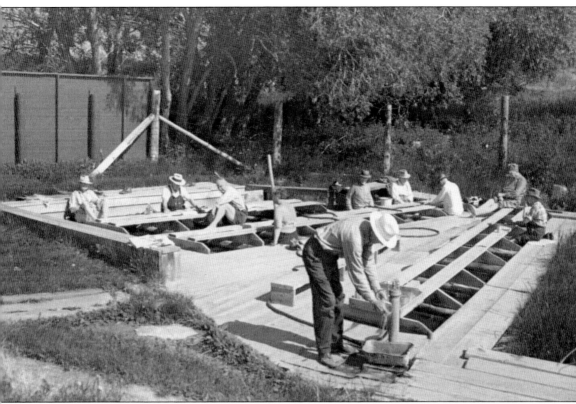

This photograph of visitors to the corn hole at Camas Hot Springs is probably from the 1950s. By this time, the hot mud pit had been expanded, and more comfortable seating had been installed. Visitors could sit across from each other with a long board "table" between them. This table allowed visitors to enjoy a game of checkers or chess with friends while they soaked their feet.

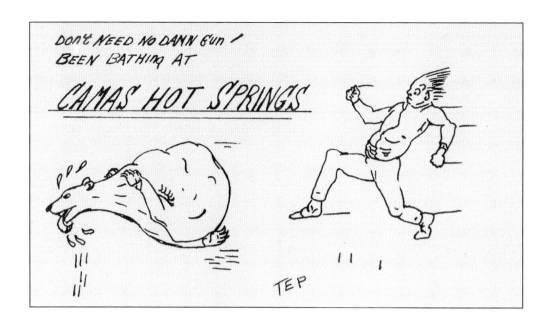

Marketing campaigns were developed to attract visitors to Camas. Visitors mailed these humorous postcards extolling the benefits of the Camas hot water to relatives and friends back home. The below postcard shows the early slogan of Camas Hot Springs: "Limp In . . . Hop Out." This slogan was later changed to "Limp In . . . Leap Out," which is now featured on a large sign at the town entrance. (Both, MHS.)

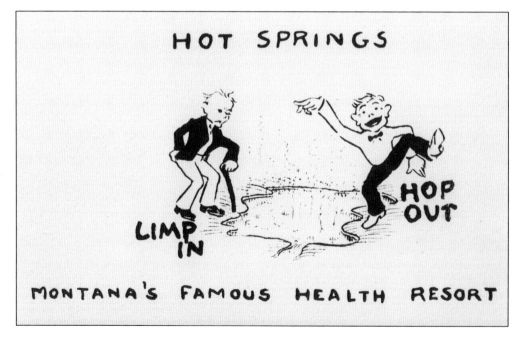

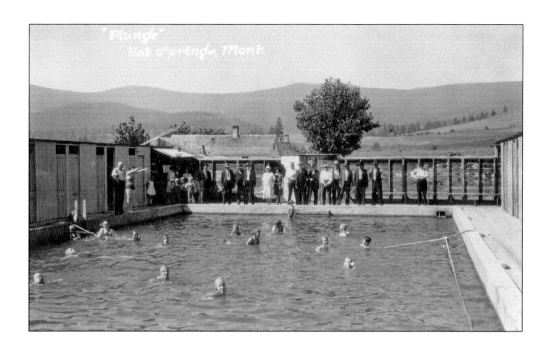

In addition to the mud pools and soaking pools at Camas Hot Springs, a mineral water plunge and swimming pool were built by the townspeople. (Both, HSM.)

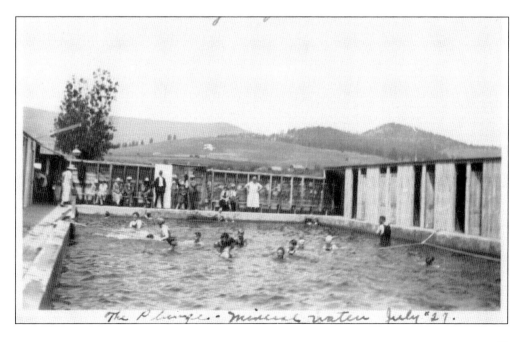

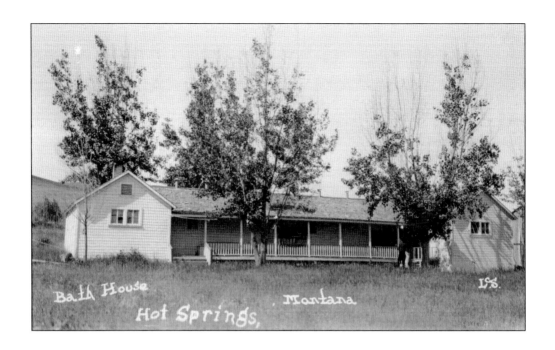

Bath House
Hot Springs, Montana
I.S.

A second bathhouse was built at Camas Hot Springs in 1913. The bathhouse had both a men's and women's section, with each containing four bathtubs. The bathhouse also contained a waiting room and a "sweat room."

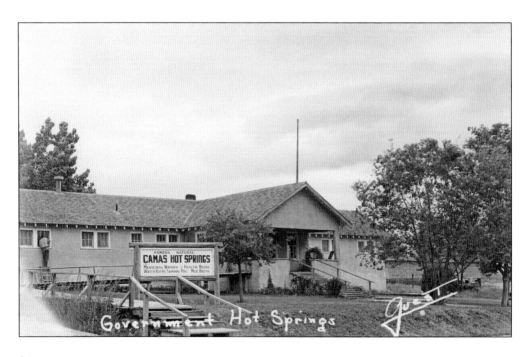

FAMOUS NATURAL
CAMAS HOT SPRINGS
MEDICINAL WATERS & HEALTH BATHS
WATER BATHS, SWIMMING POOL, MUD BATHS

Government Hot Springs

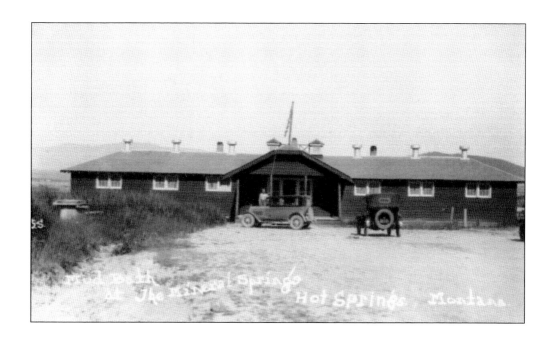

A third bathhouse was built at Camas by Al Hurst. The stucco-covered building included tub rooms and a mud bath room.

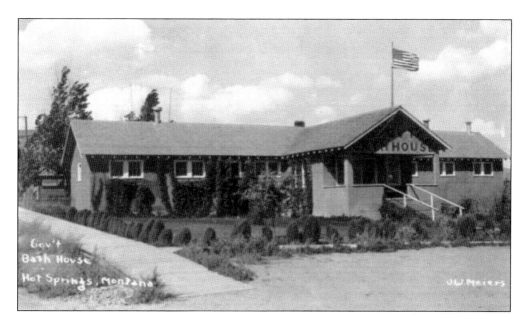

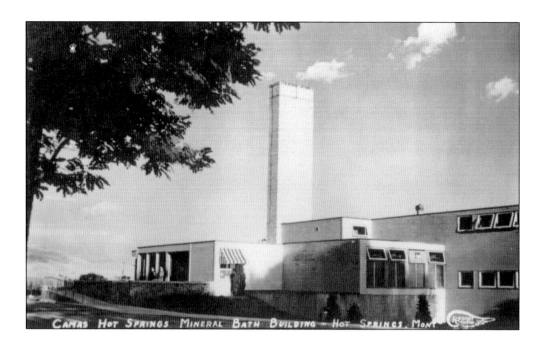

CAMAS HOT SPRINGS MINERAL BATH BUILDING - HOT SPRINGS, MONT

In 1941, the Salish and Kootenai tribes assumed ownership of the Camas Hot Springs and surrounding land, and 10 years later, they opened this large health resort named the Camas Bathhouse. The grand opening celebration and dedication were attended by Jim Thorpe, a Native American who won two gold medals in the 1912 Olympics. About 5,000 people attended the dedication. Two buffalo and two elk were barbecued, and the meat was made into sandwiches given away to the crowd.

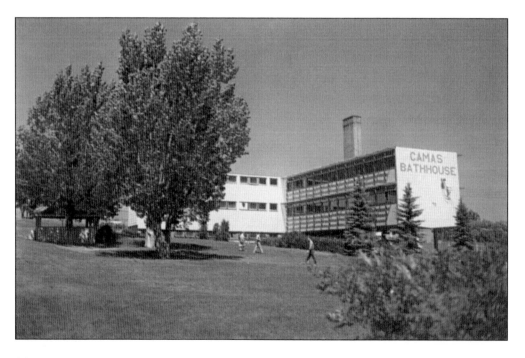

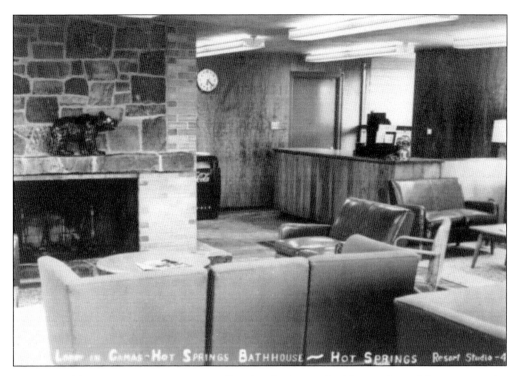

A variety of therapeutic treatments were offered at the Camas Bathhouse. One of the most popular was a three-week treatment of daily baths and mineral water consumption under the watchful eye of the Camas Bathhouse physicians. Massage therapy and steam baths were also available. The two-story facility had one floor for women and one for men.

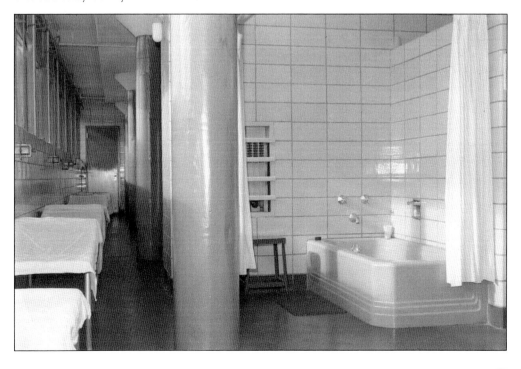

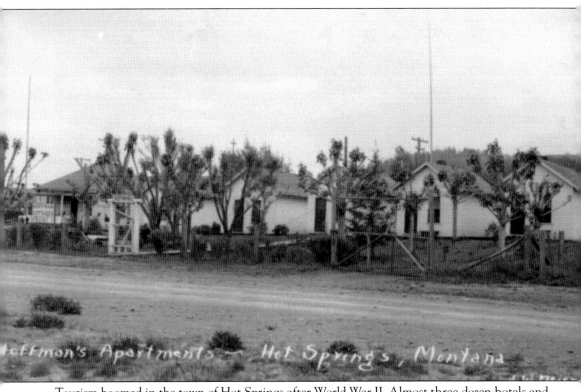

Tourism boomed in the town of Hot Springs after World War II. Almost three dozen hotels and motels were built in the town to accommodate visitors in the 1940s and 1950s. Unfortunately, the boom was short-lived, and the number of visitors dropped off in the 1960s. Many of the old hotels and motels were closed and torn down. The Camas Bathhouse closed in the late 1970s. (MHS.)

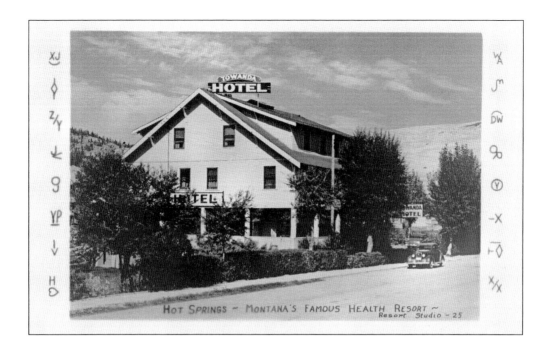

Hot Springs ~ Montana's Famous Health Resort ~
Resort Studio ~ 25

One of the most popular hotels in Hot Springs during the tourism boom of the 1940s and 1950s was the Towanda Hotel. Located just a few blocks from the Camas Bathhouse, the Towanda was in a prime location for visitors who came to Hot Springs for the popular 21-day spa treatments. (Both, MHS.)

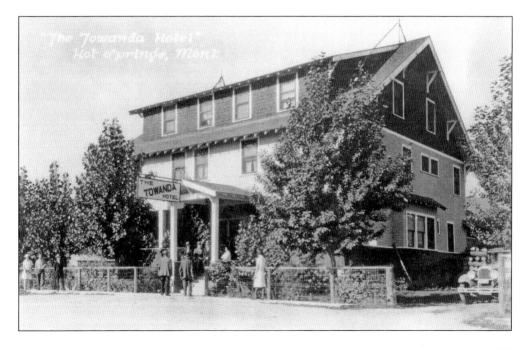

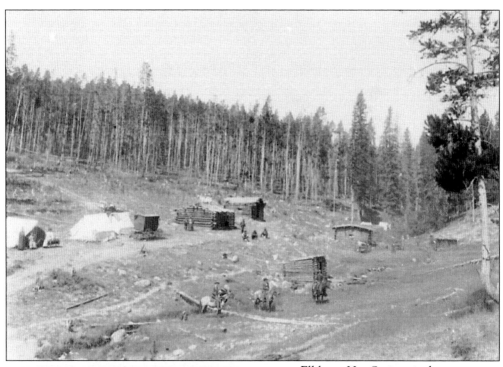

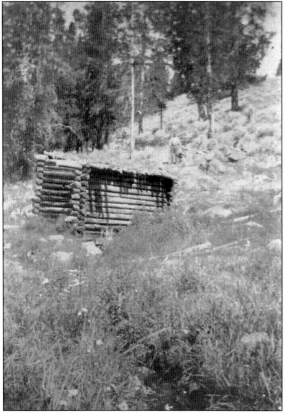

Elkhorn Hot Springs is shown here in the 1880s. A crude log bathhouse and a few log cabins were built near the springs, but many visitors camped out in tents. The hot springs were on federal land, and the federal government showed little interest in further development. In 1905, federal officials sold the rights to the hot springs to Samuel Engelsjard. Engelsjard added more cabins and a horse stable to the property. (Both, BCM.)

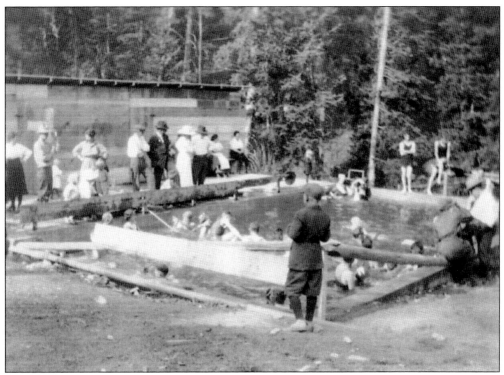

A 20-by-40-foot plunge was built at Elkhorn Hot Springs in the 1890s, followed by a second plunge that was about three times larger than the first. The original pool house was rebuilt in the 1940s after it was damaged by lightning. (Both, BCM.)

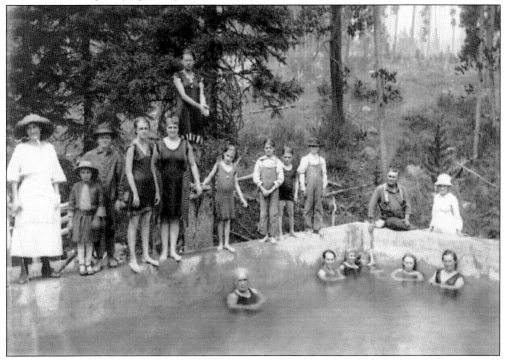

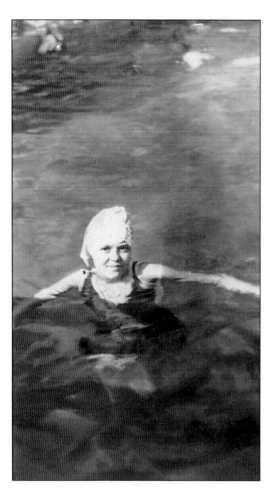

A woman wearing a bathing cap and a man in a fashionable tank top swimsuit are shown enjoying their time at the Elkhorn Hot Springs plunge around 1920. (Both, BCM.)

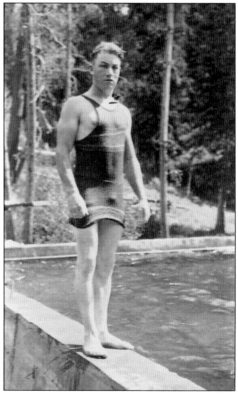

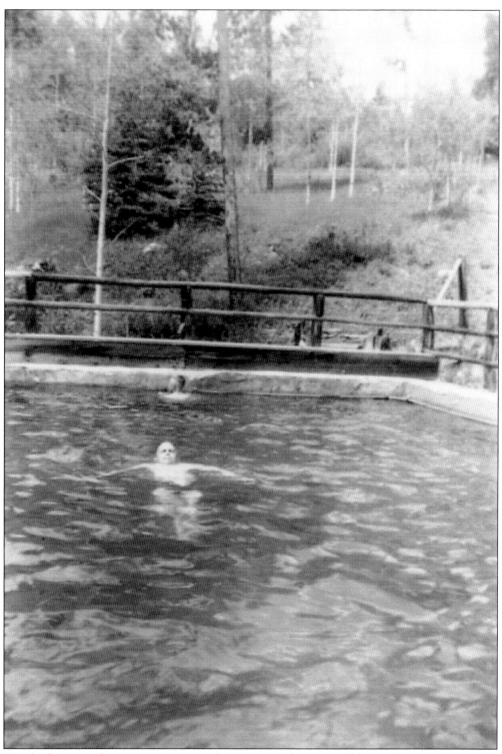

Two bathers are shown swimming in the open-air plunge at Elkhorn Hot Springs around 1920. (BCM.)

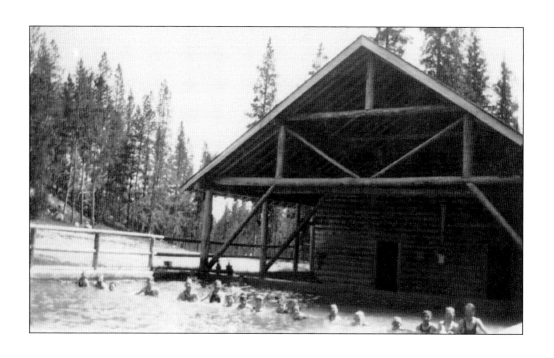

These two views of the Elkhorn Hot Springs swimming pool around 1920 show the dressing rooms and sauna. (Both, BCM.)

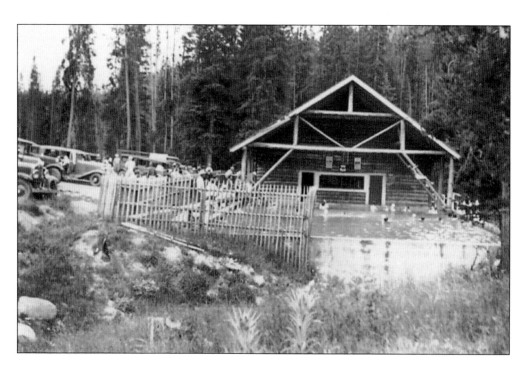

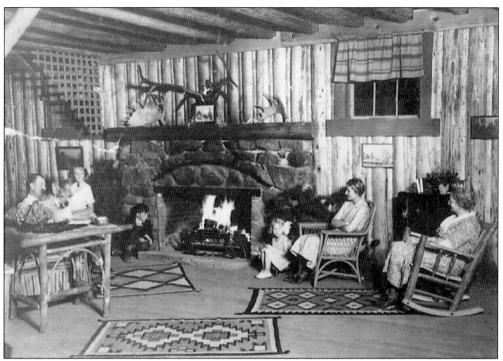

The photograph of the interior of Elkhorn Hot Springs lodge was probably taken in the 1930s. The lodge was originally built by a group of local ranchers as a private hunting retreat. (BCM.)

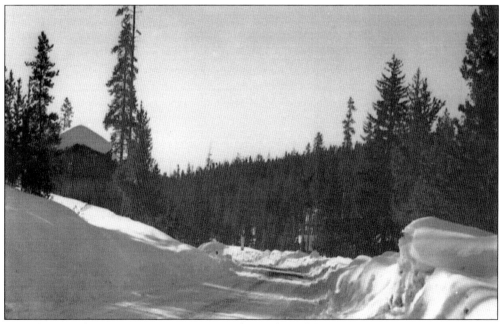

This photograph of a snowy winter scene on the road to Elkhorn Hot Springs was taken around 1925. The lodge building is on the left. (BCM.)

Gregson Hot Springs

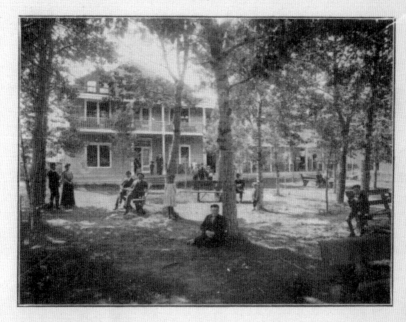
In 1869, brothers George and Eli Gregson bought a hot spring located 15 miles west of Butte from a Mr. Hulbert for the price of $60. The Gregsons built the first hotel on the property, a plunge bath, and five individual bathhouses. This hotel was destroyed by fire in 1914. The Gregsons sold the property to Milo French in 1891, but the name "Gregson Hot Springs" was used until the 1970s. This c. 1920 advertisement is promoting the resort's new two-story hotel and attached natatorium built by Milo French in 1915. Both male and female masseurs were available to guests, as well as "all kinds of private baths, vapors and small plunges and a regular sanitarium and hospital attached." By 1897, the resort hotel was heated with water from the hot springs—one of the first commercial uses of geothermal energy in Montana. (MHS.)

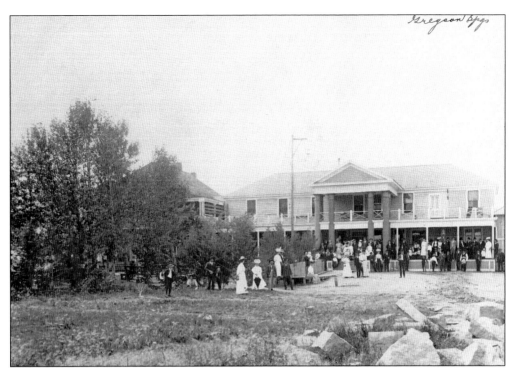

Four trains per day brought guests to Gregson Hot Springs in the early 1900s. Anaconda and Butte were full of immigrants who worked in the local smelter or deep in the underground copper mines. The resort became a gathering place for picnics on its expansive lawns during the summer months. One picnic for local miners and smelter workers attracted over 12,000 guests. The original two-story hotel built by the Gregson brothers was destroyed by fire in 1914. These two images show the second, larger hotel and natatorium built in 1915. This newer hotel also burned to the ground a little over a decade after its construction. (Both, MHS.)

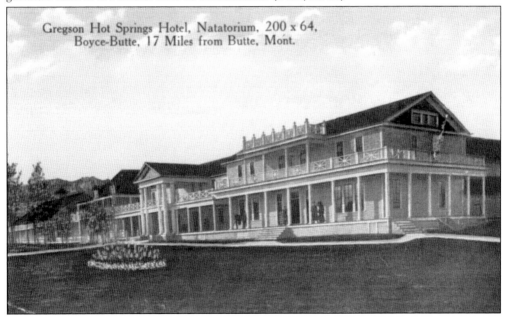

Gregson Hot Springs Hotel, Natatorium, 200 x 64,
Boyce-Butte, 17 Miles from Butte, Mont.

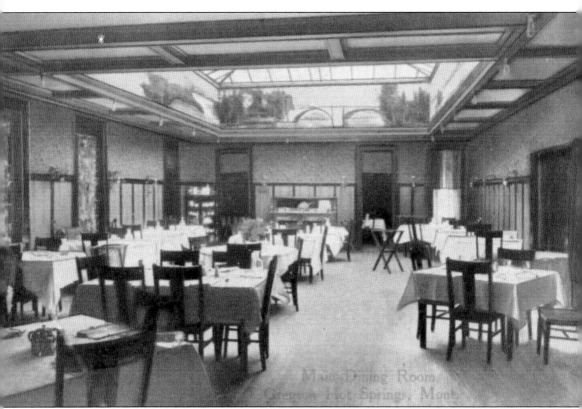

The elegant dining room in the Gregson Hot Springs Hotel is pictured here around 1928. Locally produced meats and vegetables were served to hotel guests. The mineral water from the hot springs also may have been on the menu. According to an article in the *Butte Daily Miner,* "The water has not an unpleasant taste to some, however it may taste to others. It is said that by seasoning it with pepper and salt it makes a very palatable soup. When drank as hot as can be borne, the taste of sulphur is pronounced enough to lead one to the conclusion that his Satanic Majesty superintends the brewing in a branch kitchen just below."

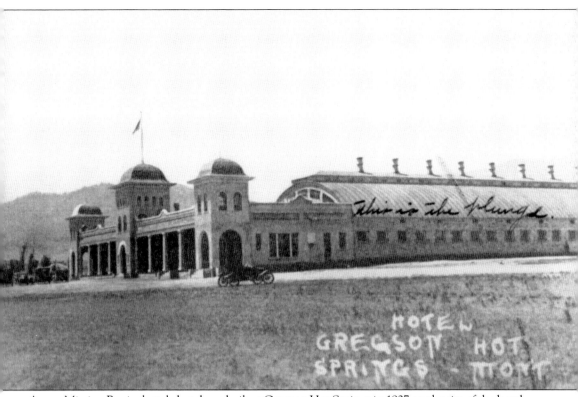

A new Mission Revival–style hotel was built at Gregson Hot Springs in 1927 on the site of the hotel that had burned in 1925. The *Anaconda Standard* called the new hotel and plunge "the Saratoga of the Northwest." The resort included a 65-by-195-foot warm-water plunge as well as a cold-water pool adjacent to the plunge. Guests were encouraged to alternate bathing in the hot water and the cold water, producing an invigorating effect on the skin and body. The enclosed indoor pool was surrounded by slides, chutes, springboards, and high-diving platforms. A dance pavilion was built on the second floor of the entrance to the resort, with the dance floor made of maple. Community dances with live music were often held there, attracting large crowds. (MHS.)

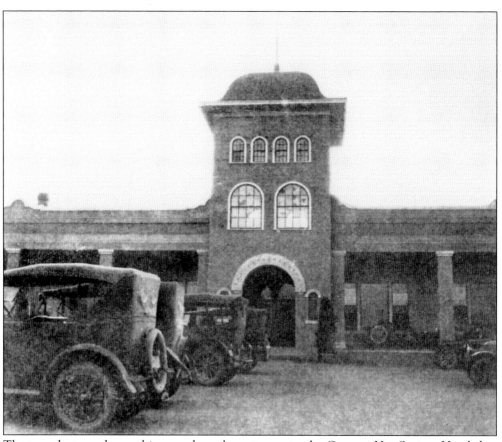

The two photographs on this page show the entrance to the Gregson Hot Springs Hotel that was built in 1927. The hotel and plunge eventually fell into disrepair, and the resort was closed in 1971. That same year, a Canadian firm purchased the property; the firm built a new hotel and pool called Fairmont Hot Springs Resort, which is still in operation today. (Both, MHS.)

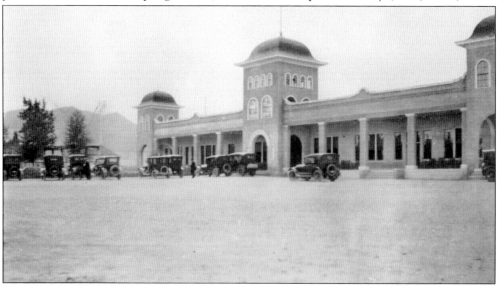

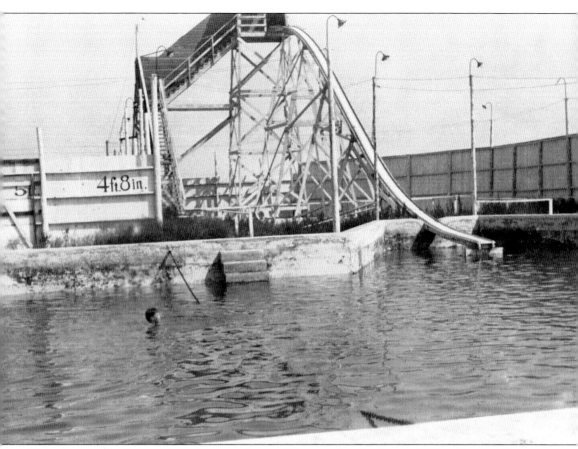

This photograph of an outdoor plunge and waterslide was taken in August 1929 at Gregson Hot Springs. (MHS.)

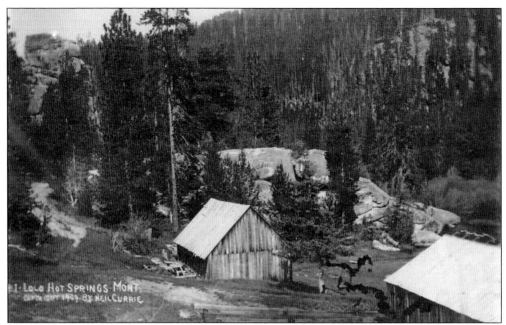

In 1885, Fred Lemke purchased Lolo Hot Springs and the surrounding land. Lemke built a small resort complete with a hotel, a dining room, cabins, a saloon, and a store. William Boyle purchased the resort from Fred Lemke in 1888. Missoula was only 40 miles east of the hot springs, and many Missoula residents vacationed at the little resort, although the journey was difficult. Boyle provided a stagecoach to bring guests to Lolo Hot Springs, charging $5 per person. A fire destroyed the hotel in 1903, and Boyle sold the land and hot springs to Paul Gerber. Gerber increased the size of the resort to 400 acres. Lolo Hot Springs became a popular destination for tent campers, with more than 500 tents surrounding the hot springs on some holiday weekends. These photographs show the Lolo resort and bathhouse around 1909. (Both, RCM.)

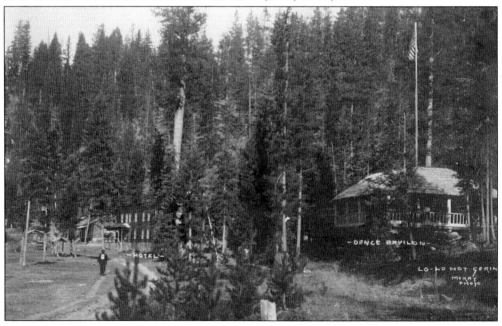

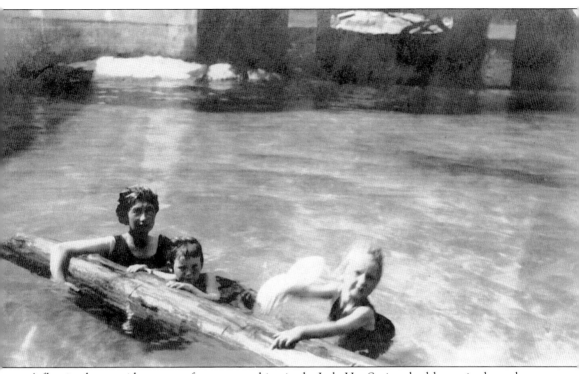

A floating log provides support for guests soaking in the Lolo Hot Springs bathhouse in the early 1900s. (HMFM.)

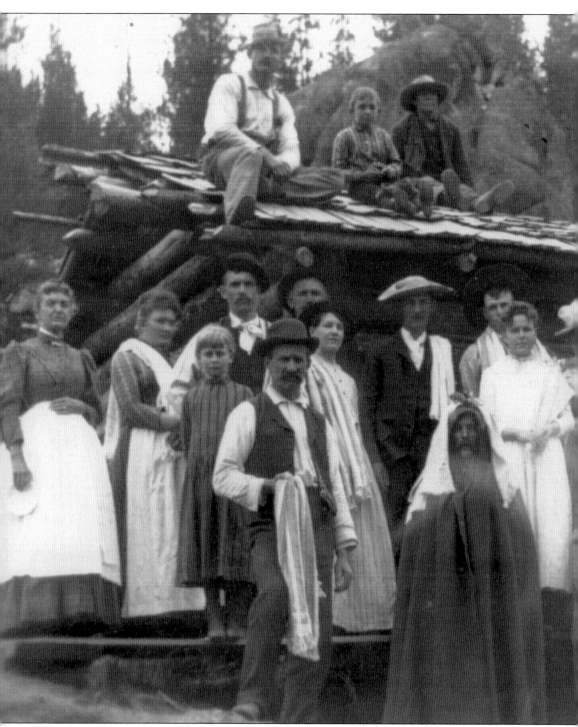

This group of soakers is shown relaxing outside the bathhouse at Lolo Hot Springs around 1900. Many of them are bundled in towels or blankets after their soak. Explorers Meriwether Lewis and William Clark described Lolo Hot Springs in their journals during their trek across the country. Clark recorded in 1806 that he "bathed and remained in 10 minutes. It was with difficulty I

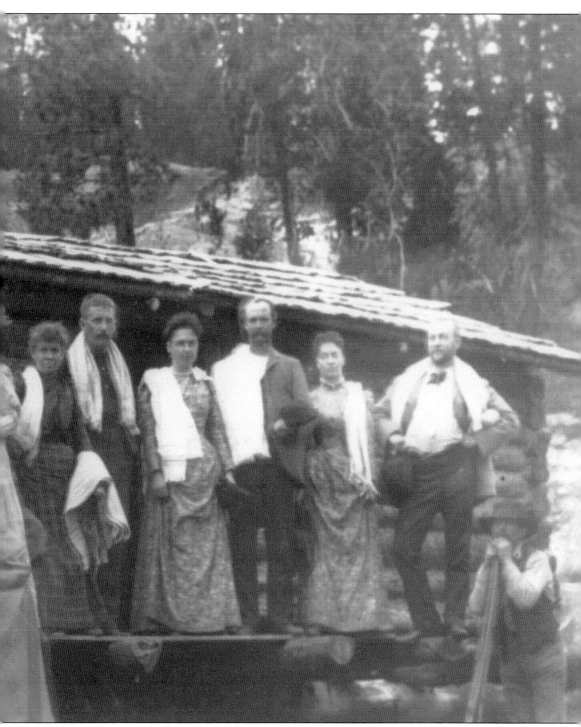

could remain this long and it caused a profuse sweat. Two other bold springs adjacent to this are much warmer, their heat being so great as to make the hand of a person smart extremely when immersed." (UM.)

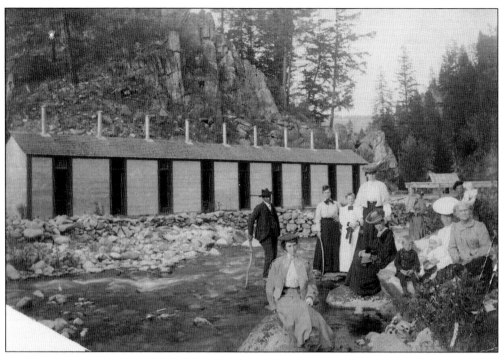

In 1883, Ed Wiles of Stevensville visited Medicine Hot Springs, about 80 miles south of Missoula, to see if the hot water would relieve his rheumatism. He was pleased with the results and filed a homestead on the land surrounding the springs. Wiles built a bathhouse in 1895. The bathhouse had nine compartments, each with a large wooden tub sunk to ground level. (RCM.)

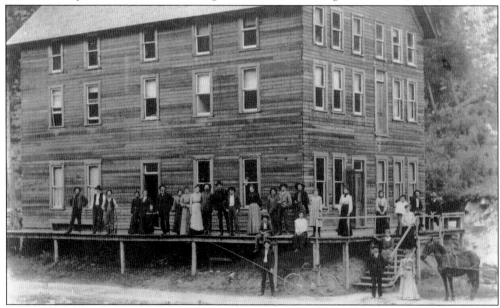

In 1895, Ed Wiles partnered with Dr. George Lord to build a hotel across the river from the hot springs. The three-story hotel had 25 rooms. This photograph shows a boy in front of the hotel with a fly rod and bicycle. Guests could walk a few steps from the hotel to Warm Springs Creek, where they could cast a fly into the creek to catch a trout for supper. (RCM.)

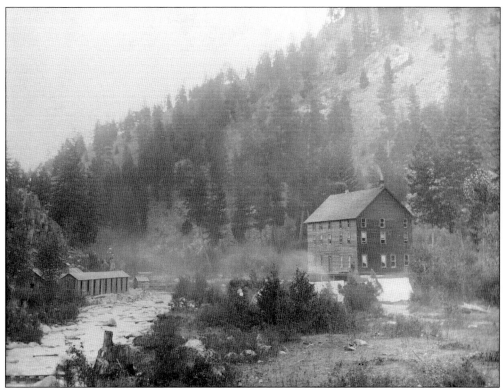

An upstream view from 1896 shows the Medicine Hot Springs bathhouse on one side of Warm Springs Creek and the hotel on the other side. The hotel was torn down by owner Ed Smith after he purchased the property in 1910. Three generations of the Smith family managed the resort—Ed Smith, his son Barton, and his grandson Tom. (RCM.)

In 1912, a Mr. Page built the second bathhouse at Medicine Springs for new owner Ed Smith. This photograph shows the plunge during a Fourth of July celebration around 1920. Every hour, the hot springs produced about 6,000 gallons of 120-degree water, which was mixed with cold spring water and used to fill the pool. (RCM.)

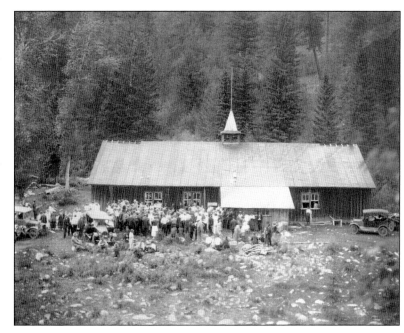

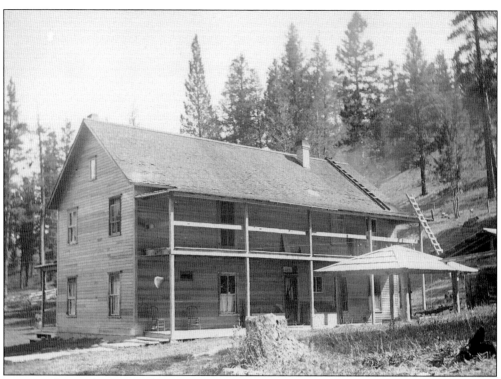

Ninety miles south of Missoula, in the Bitterroot Valley, Gallogly Springs flows out of a hillside at 110 degrees Fahrenheit. This two-story 14-room hotel was built near the springs in 1896 by Frank Allen, who sold the property to James Gallogly a year later. The hotel was torn down in 1941, and a new outdoor pool was constructed on the former site of the hotel. The Northern Pacific Railway produced advertisements promoting the resort in the 1930s and 1940s. The property remained in the Gallogly family until the 1970s. (Both, RCM.)

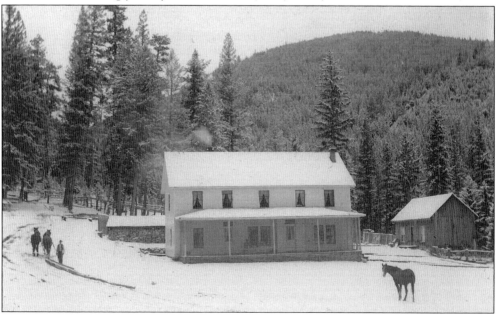

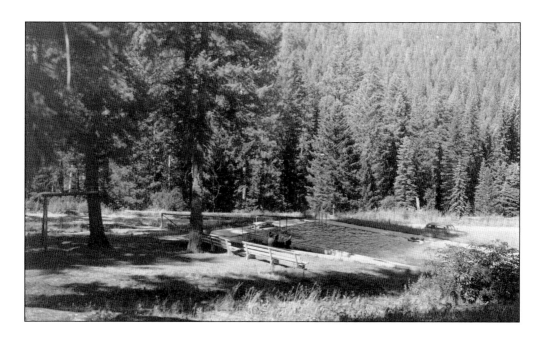

The above image shows the Gallogly Springs swimming pool in the late 1930s. The below image shows the newer pool built in 1941. This newer swimming pool consisted of a 25-by-40-foot cement plunge with "under-water lights for night swimming." The plunge was enclosed by a glass wall to keep out cold winds. A two-story building at the north end of the pool contained a kitchen and dining room, as well as dressing rooms and showers for bathers. The dining room could hold up to 60 adults. F.G. Moore leased and managed the springs in the 1940s. (Above, RCM; below, MHS.)

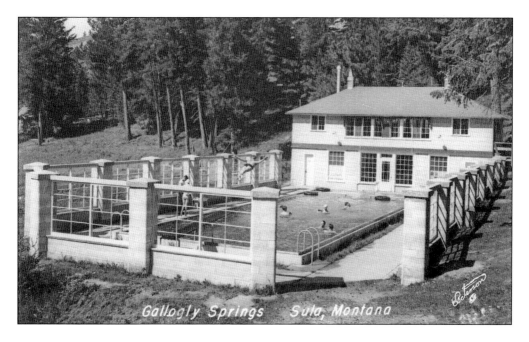

Gallogly Springs   Sula, Montana

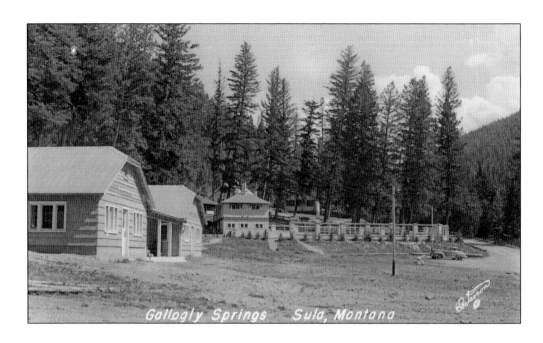

During the 1940s, Gallogly Springs was often leased out for months at a time to 4-H clubs and other youth groups. A guest lodge with sleeping quarters was built to accommodate these groups. The H-shaped lodge also contained meeting rooms. In front of the lodge was a shallow basin that was filled with water in the winter, creating an ice rink. A street lamp in the center of the rink provided lighting for night skating. Ten guest cabins were also built nearby. Winter guests would often combine a visit to the hot springs with a day of snow skiing at Lost Trail Pass, located about five miles south of the resort. (Both, MHS.)

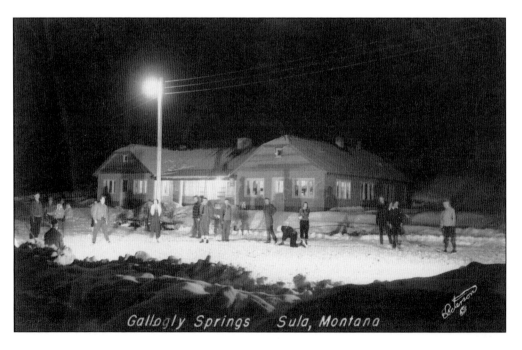

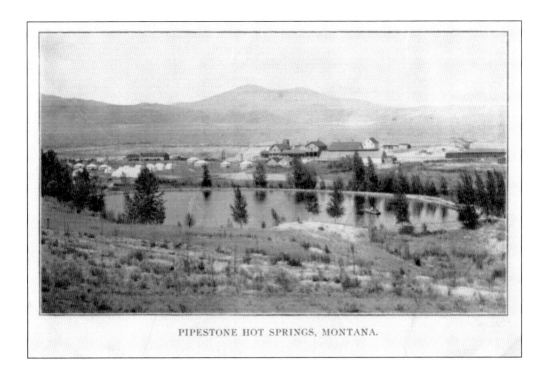

PIPESTONE HOT SPRINGS, MONTANA.

Pipestone Hot Springs, located about 20 miles east of Butte, were developed in 1878 by John Paul. In 1912, John Alley, an attorney for the Anaconda Mining Company in Butte, purchased the hot springs and surrounding land. The Alley family continues to own the property to this day. Approximately 100 canvas-roofed guest cabins were built on the resort grounds. The facilities included a vapor bathhouse, hot-mud soaking, and a 25-by-100-foot warm-water swimming pool.

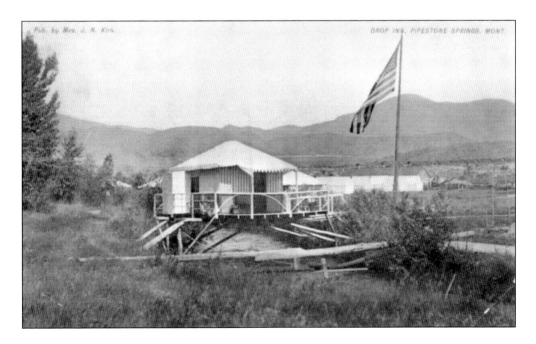

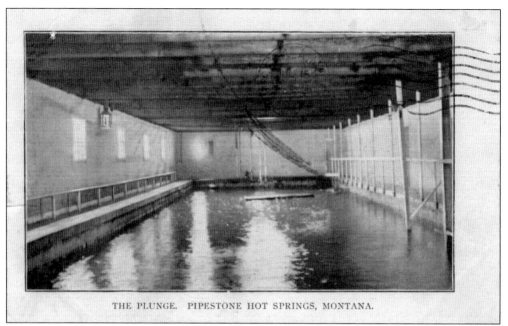

THE PLUNGE. PIPESTONE HOT SPRINGS, MONTANA.

The water at Pipestone Hot Springs was praised for its medicinal value. An 1887 article in the *Butte Holiday Intermountain* observed that invalids "suffering from rheumatism, neuralgia, dyspepsia, paralysis, kidney and liver complaints, impure blood, lead poisoning, etc., experienced speedy and permanent relief after a course of bathing and drinking."

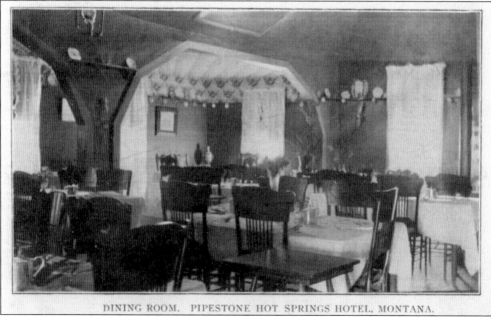

DINING ROOM. PIPESTONE HOT SPRINGS HOTEL, MONTANA.

The dining room in one of Pipestone's early hotels is shown in this photograph. The first hotel at Pipestone burned to the ground in 1913. The hotel was rebuilt, but the new hotel also succumbed to fire in 1918. Only a player piano and some furniture were saved in the blaze that destroyed the second hotel. The resort continued attracting guests until 1963, when the Alley family closed it to the public.

Fifty miles west of Bozeman, Potosi Hot Springs is one of the few hot springs in Montana located high in a mountain range instead of in a valley. The hot springs were claimed by Horace Walter in 1892. Walter constructed a large hotel, greenhouse, swimming pool, and bathhouse near the springs, which attracted gold miners from the nearby town of Pony. The dining room (pictured below) in the hotel served meals to hungry travelers after a soak and swim in the hot springs. About two miles farther up the mountain road sat a public bathhouse atop another hot spring (pictured at right). In 1902, Walter sold his property to William Young from Butte, who operated the resort until it was abandoned in 1909. (Right, MHS.)

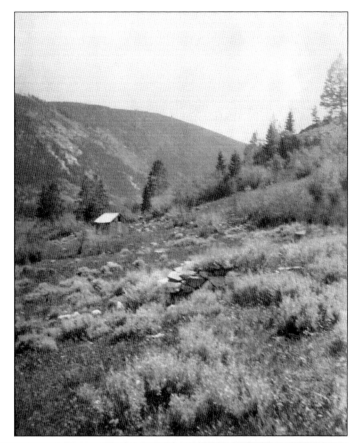

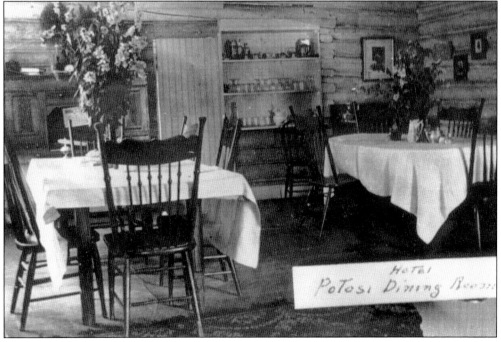

Hotel Potosi Dining Room

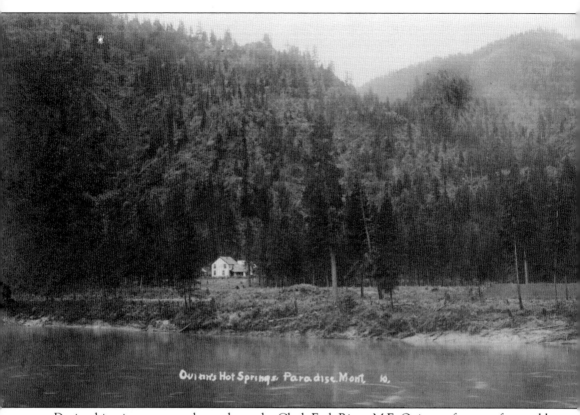

Quinn's Hot Springs, Paradise, Mont. 10.

During his trips on an ore barge down the Clark Fork River, M.E. Quinn, a foreman for a gold mine about 20 miles east of St. Regis, noticed Native Americans bathing in a hot spring. Quinn filed a homestead on the springs in the late 1880s and developed a small hotel and soaking pool on the property. Quinn provided guests with opportunities for horseback riding, hunting, and fishing in addition to soaking. The *Weekly Plainsman* reported in 1896 on the "remarkably efficacious hot springs owned by M.E. Quinn, which have effected surprising cures in rheumatic and kidney diseases, and are fast becoming a popular summer and winter resort." (MHS.)

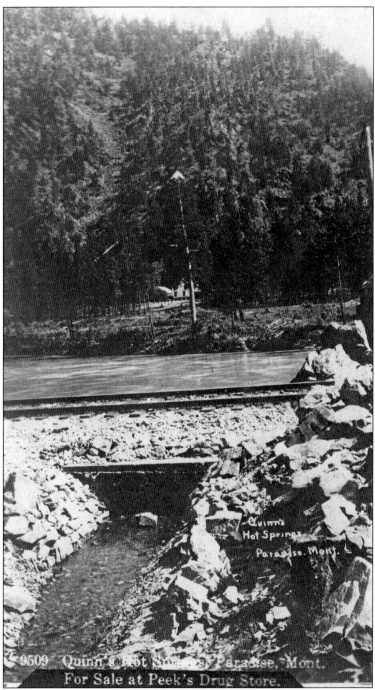

Quinn's
Hot Springs
Paradise. Mont.

9509 Quinn's Hot Springs, Paradise, Mont.
For Sale at Peek's Drug Store.

In the early days of M.E. Quinn's resort, no road was available to transport tourists. Resort visitors had to either float down the Clark Fork River or hike over the mountain ridge behind the resort to reach the hot springs. By 1909, a railroad had been built along the river across from the resort. Quinn built a swinging bridge across the river between his resort and the rail line, and trains would stop at the bridge to drop off and pick up resort visitors. Quinn would greet visitors at the train, load their luggage into a wheelbarrow, and lead them across the bridge to the resort. (MHS.)

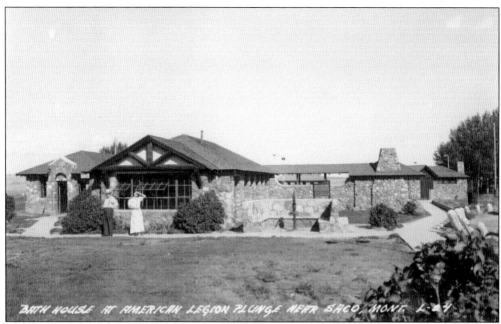

A well driller near the north central Montana town of Malta struck a large volume of hot water while drilling for oil in 1924. The well produced over 700 gallons per minute of artesian water with a temperature near 105 degrees Fahrenheit. A local rancher built a small enclosure around the well in 1927, and nearby residents would gather to bathe in the warm water. In the 1930s, a new resort was developed with funding from the federal government's Works Progress Administration enacted by Pres. Franklin Roosevelt. Roosevelt himself was a proponent of the use of hot water for treating illness and had often bathed at Warm Springs, Georgia, to help relieve his polio symptoms. The owners of the resort employed experienced stonemasons to construct this beautiful bathhouse and other buildings as part of the new resort, which was named the American Legion Health Plunge. The name was later changed to the Sleeping Buffalo Resort.

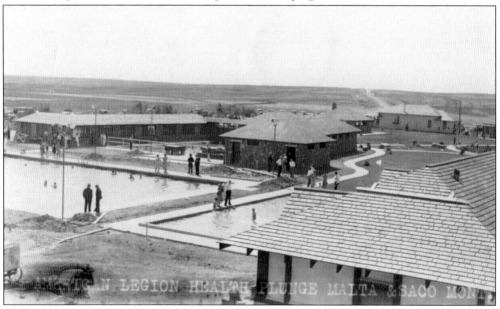

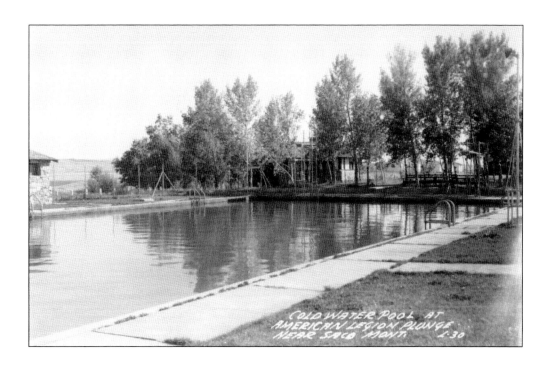

From the early 1930s until 1957, the American Legion Health Plunge (later called the Sleeping Buffalo Resort) thrived near Malta, with both cold- and warm-water swimming pools available to guests. In 1957, the flow of water to the resort abruptly stopped when the well casing collapsed more than 1,000 feet below the ground surface. The resort was closed for over a year and a half until a new well was drilled and water once again flowed into the bathing pools.

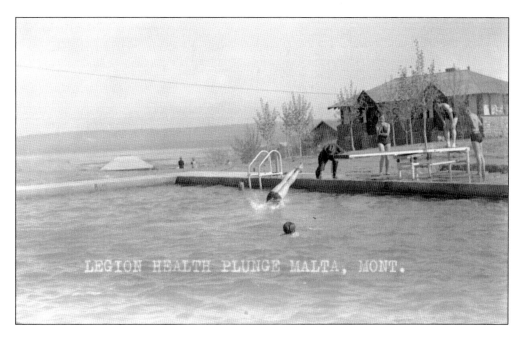

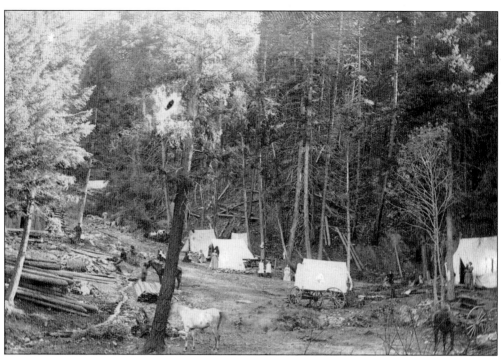

In the late 1880s, visitors to Sleeping Child Hot Springs camped in tents and cooked their own food. A stagecoach from Hamilton would bring food and mail to the campers about twice a week. Besides soaking in the mineral waters of Sleeping Child, visitors often engaged in hunting. One visitor reported in 1892 that he had "succeeded in killing two grizzly bears, three deer, and twenty grouse." He left the hot springs with two wagons loaded down with the animals.

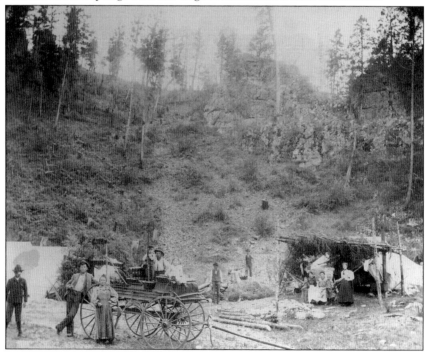

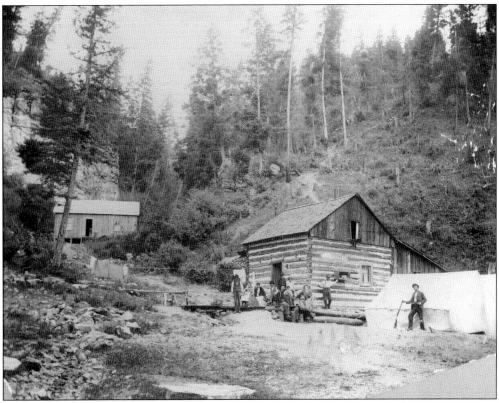

The first person to claim the land around Sleeping Child Hot Springs was William Real, in 1889. Sleeping Child Hot Springs may have been named after a Native American legend. According to the legend, a mother and child were fleeing from a warring tribe, and the mother hid her child near the hot springs. Upon returning later that evening, the mother found her child sleeping peacefully, lulled into slumber by the murmuring of the hot springs. (Both, RCM.)

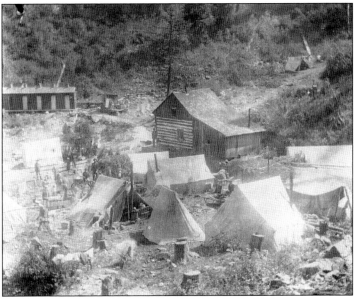

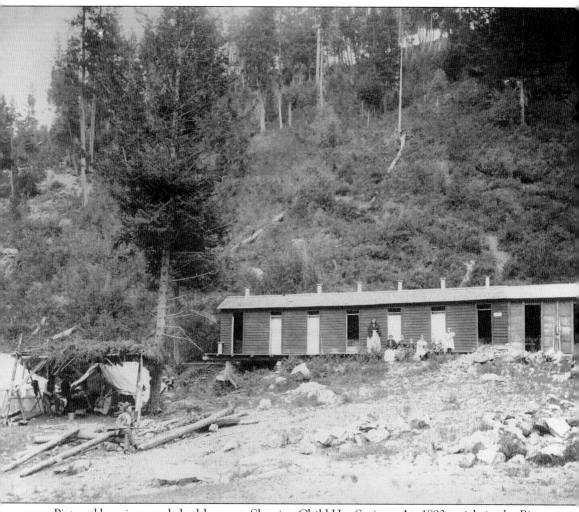

Pictured here is an early bathhouse at Sleeping Child Hot Springs. An 1892 article in the *Bitter Root Bugle* extolled the curative power of the hot water: "Venereal diseases and rheumatism in all its varied form, speedily yield to the magic medicinal properties of these remarkable hot waters which gush forth from nature's bosom." (RCM.)

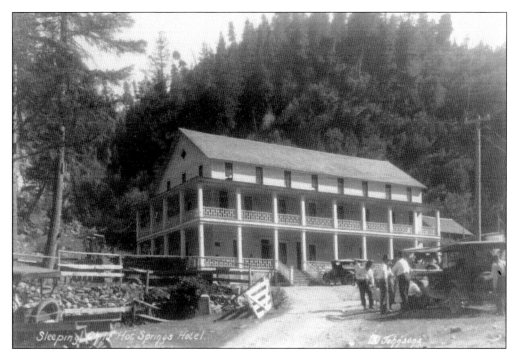

The three-story Sleeping Child Resort Hotel (above) was built in 1917 by B.F. Heavilin. The hotel had 25 rooms, a large lobby with a pool table, electric lights, and heat provided by the geothermal water piped in from the hot spring and circulated through radiators. Heavilin also built a large plunge (below) across the road from the hotel in 1922. Heavilin sold the resort to H. Blybert of Missoula in 1931. (Both, UM.)

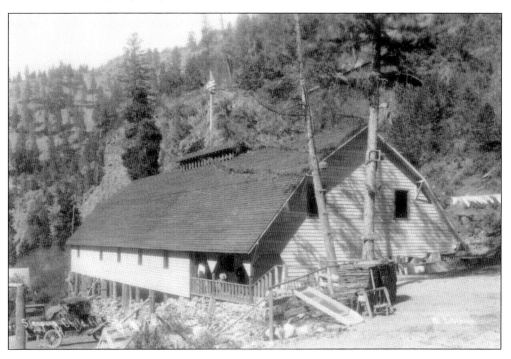

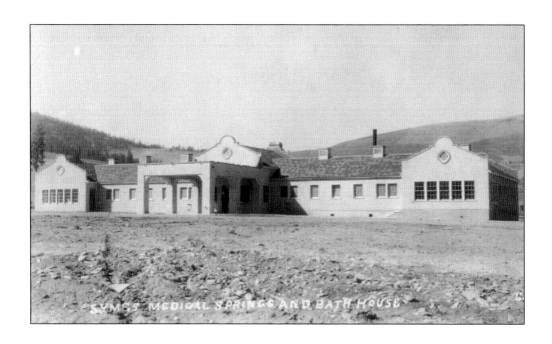

Built by Kiva and Fred Symes in 1928 in the town of Hot Springs, the Symes Hotel prospered from the boom in tourists who arrived to take advantage of the many thermal water opportunities. The hotel featured indoor soaking tubs off the lobby entrance, as well as a sunroom with special "vita glass" that admitted only "healthful" solar rays. The hotel was owned by the Symes family until the early 1990s.

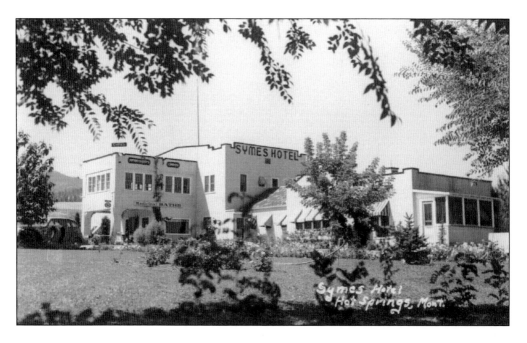

Pictured here is an advertisement for the Symes Hotel and its medicinal waters. Another Symes advertisement told the story of an elderly man who traveled to Symes every year to bathe in the hot water. "Maybe it's a sign of old age," he said, "but if it is, all the more reason I should grow old as young as possible."

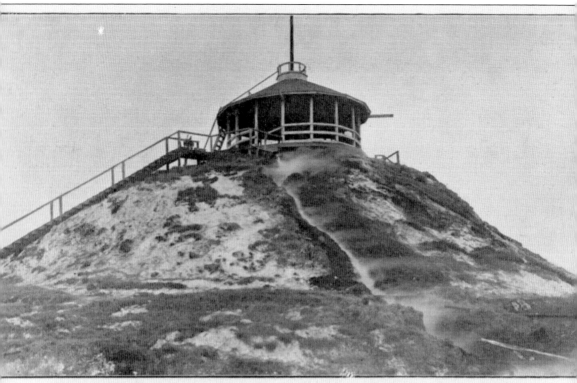

"The Mound," Montana State Hospital, Warm Springs, Mont., 180° F.

Twenty miles west of Butte, a 40-foot-tall mound of calcium carbonate, stained brown by iron deposits in the hot water gurgling from the mound's apex, rose from the valley floor. The thermal waters were simply named "Warm Springs." Early explorers who viewed the mound from a distance thought that it was the lodge of a Native American tribe. (The nearby town of Deer Lodge got its name from observers who saw deer grazing near the hot springs mound and called it "the deer's lodge.") Louis Belanger built the first bathhouse near the mound in 1867. The state of Montana eventually acquired the property and built the Montana State Hospital adjacent to the Warm Springs mound.

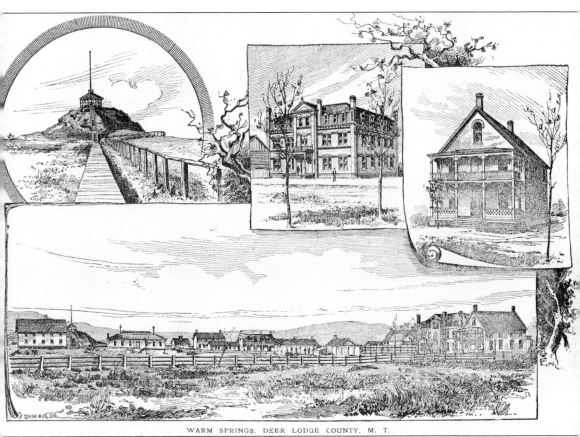

WARM SPRINGS, DEER LODGE COUNTY, M. T.

Dr. Charles F. Mussingbrod and Dr. A. Mitchell purchased the Warm Springs property from Louis Belanger in 1877 and acquired a state contract to house Montana's mental patients. The partners operated both a health resort and the mental hospital on the same property, with three plunge baths—one for male patients, a second plunge for female patients, and a third plunge for resort guests. The construction of the buildings and grounds was designed to keep the patients and resort guests separated. A local paper, the *Rocky Mountain Husbandman*, observed in 1885 that "so complete is the construction of the buildings and grounds that while sixty insane persons are accommodated in the asylum, visitors sojourning for health or pleasure are in no way disturbed." Mussingbrod and Mitchell were paid $1 per patient per day to provide care.

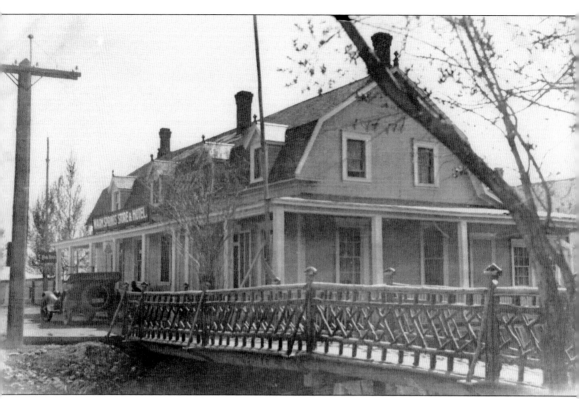

The Warm Springs Hotel was torn down in the 1990s during a major construction period for the mental hospital.

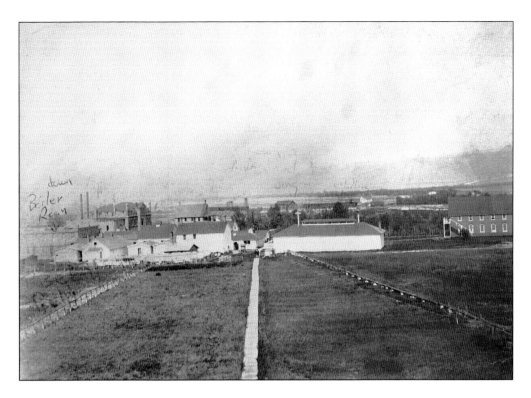

In 1912, the Montana legislature purchased the mental institution from Dr. Charles F. Mussingbrod and Dr. A. Mitchell and renamed it the Montana State Hospital. The hospital expanded through the decades, adding dormitories and specialized treatment and rehabilitation buildings to the property. At its peak period in the 1950s, the hospital housed over 2,000 patients per year.

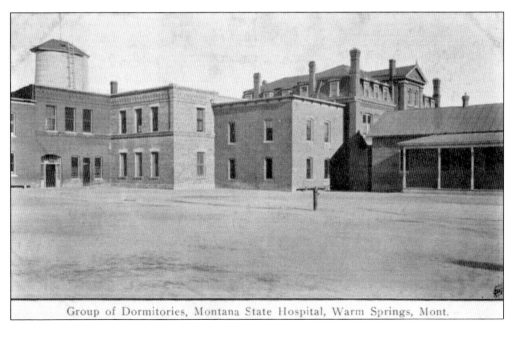

Group of Dormitories, Montana State Hospital, Warm Springs, Mont.

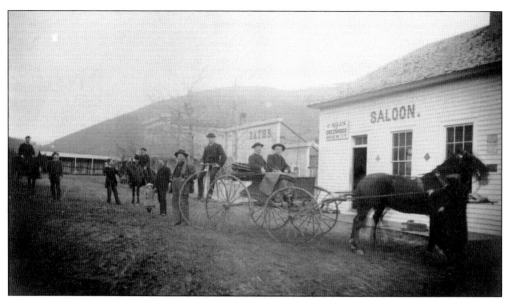

Ferdinand J. Wassweiler arrived in the Helena area in 1865, purchasing 160 acres of land and a hot spring about 10 miles west of town. By 1866, he had established Wassweiler's Hot Springs Resort on the property, complete with a bathhouse and a saloon. A local newspaper, *The Montana Radiator*, wrote that the hot springs provided "Health for the afflicted—if any of our readers wish to enjoy health, strength, longevity and prosperity, they should try a visit to the Hot Springs. . . . These springs are the cure-all of the present age. It matters not what your disease is after washing in these life-giving waters you are bound to come out with a clean skin. . . . The proprietor can satisfy the most incredulous that a great number of cases of Inflammatory Rheumatism have been cured by the use of the Hot Springs." (Both, MHS.)

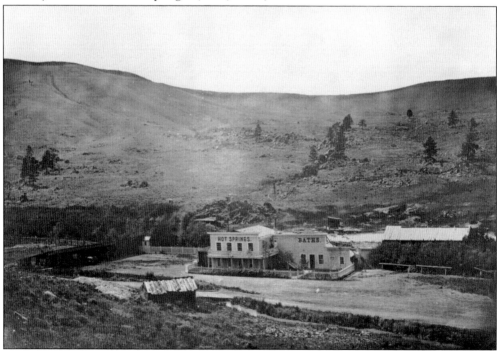

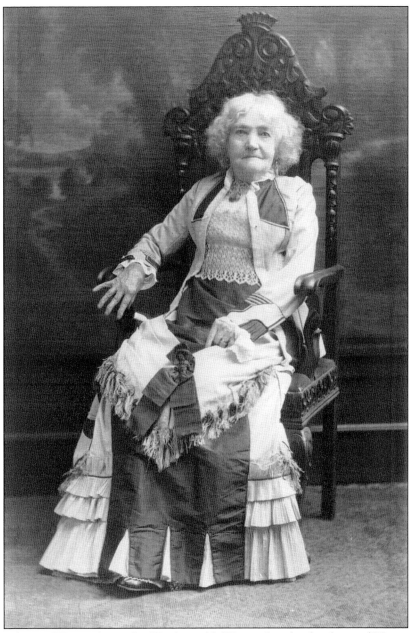

This is Catherine Wassweiler, wife of Ferdinand J. Wassweiler, the developer of Wassweiler Hot Springs. Catherine and Ferdinand were married in Fort Leavenworth, Kansas, in 1864. Within a year of their marriage, the Wassweilers had moved to Helena. A decade after establishing their first hot springs business, the Wassweilers sold the resort and a portion of the land and water rights to Charles A. Broadwater, who built the fabulous Broadwater Hot Springs Resort in 1889 (see pages 96–105). Ferdinand built a second bathhouse and hotel in 1883 on the remaining land. The second hotel featured seven exterior doors that connected to seven separate rooms for guests. The bathhouse had four rooms, each containing wooden soaking tubs. This second Wassweiler resort was well known for its delicious chicken dinners. Ferdinand's failing health forced him to close the resort in 1904. Ferdinand died in 1908, and Catherine died in 1924. (MHS.)

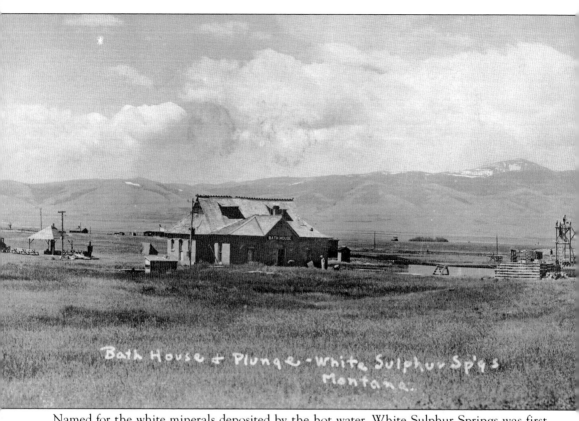

Bath House & Plunge - White Sulphur Sp'gs Montana.

Named for the white minerals deposited by the hot water, White Sulphur Springs was first commercialized in 1872 by James Brewer. Brewer built a 12-by-12-foot plunge over the springs. Dr. William Parberry bought the water rights to the springs from Brewer in 1877 and expanded the development, adding two more pools, a dressing room, and an administration building. The *Rocky Mountain Husbandman*, the local newspaper, often wrote articles about the small resort praising its medical benefits and keeping track of out-of-town visitors. (MHS.)

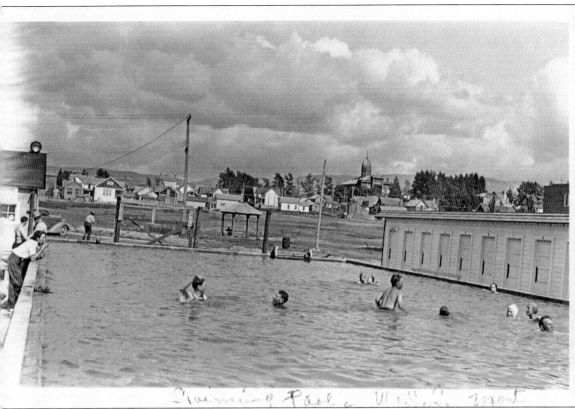

A new outdoor pool and small motel were built in the 1950s at White Sulphur Springs. The spring water was high in sulfates, and a "rotten egg" smell was noticeable. The owners of the resort praised the benefits of the sulphurous water and said soaking in the pools left a bather's skin silky smooth. (MHS.)

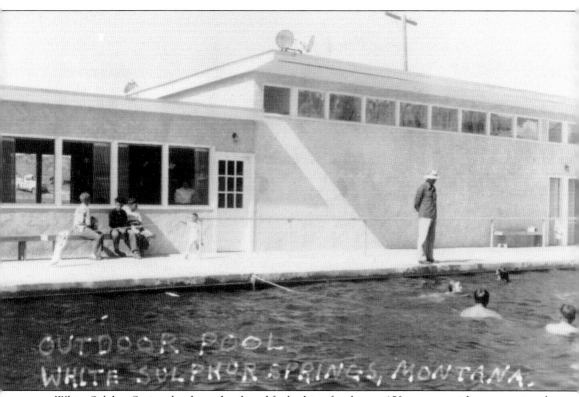

OUTDOOR POOL
WHITE SULPHUR SPRINGS, MONTANA.

White Sulphur Springs has been developed for bathing for close to 150 years, providing recreational opportunities to generations of area residents. The resort has been extensively remodeled over the years and presently includes a motel and medical clinic.

Three

ELEGANT QUEENS— MONTANA'S GRAND RESORTS

A handful of Montana's hot springs were realizations of the visions of immigrants who had fond memories of the palatial European spas they had left behind— elegant hotels, sumptuous meals, and breathtaking natatoriums and soaking parlors where travelers could indulge their taste for culture and refinement. In the early 1900s, the grandest of Montana resorts offered visitors a standard of luxury more commonly found in larger cities on the East Coast. The hot springs resorts in Montana that occupied this rarified upper echelon include Chico Hot Springs, Broadwater Hot Springs, Boulder Hot Springs, and Corwin Hot Springs. The hotel at Broadwater Hot Springs is shown in the photograph at right. (MHS.)

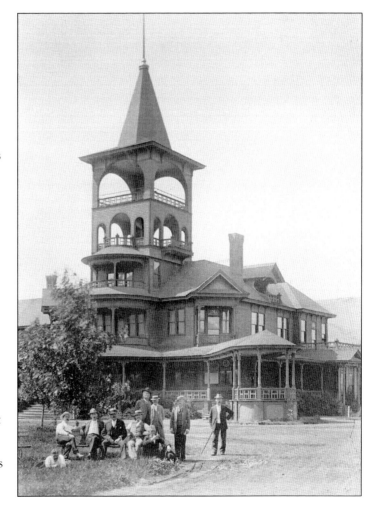

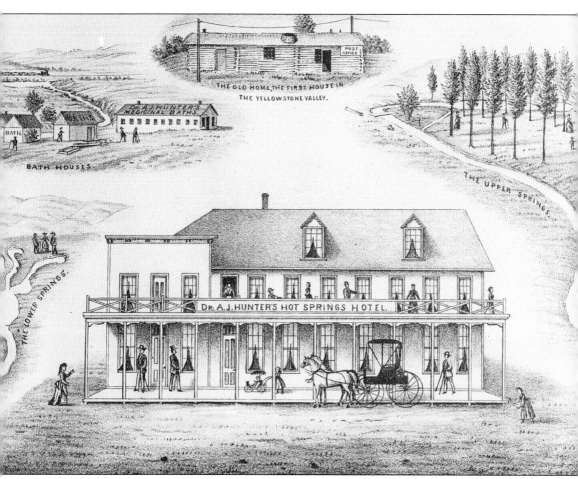

Dr. A.J. Hunter filed a claim on Hunter's Hot Springs east of Livingston in the 1860s and built a two-story wood-frame hotel on the property in 1883. Prior to the hotel construction, both Crow Indians and early settlers frequented the hot springs. Dr. Hunter reported seeing at least 1,000 Indian teepees around the hot springs during his first visit.

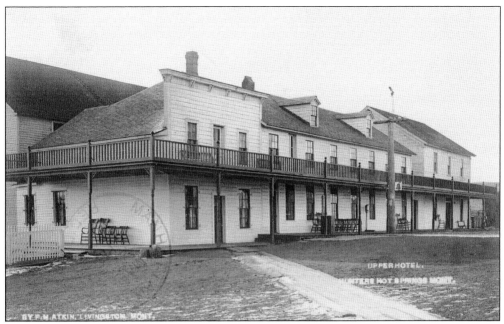

Pictured above is the original hotel that existed at Hunter's Hot Springs prior to the building of the Hotel Dakota in 1909. The below photograph shows the same hotel in June 1898 with a stagecoach in front. A cold-water spring located about a half-mile from the upper hotel was a popular destination for guests on an evening walk. (Above, UM; below, YGM.)

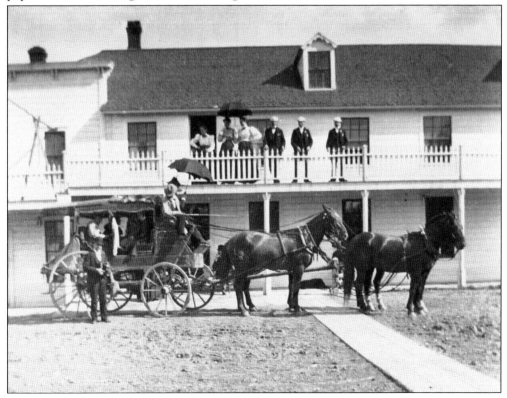

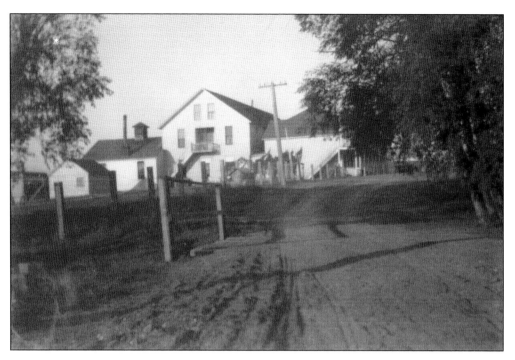

This is a c. 1885 view of Dr. A.J. Hunter's Hot Springs Hotel. Dr. Hunter touted the miraculous healing properties of the natural hot springs, including a cure for baldness in men. Dr. Hunter also claimed that his hot springs location was one of only four in the world that contained a measurable electric current. This original hotel was converted to an administration office space once the new Hotel Dakota was built in 1909. (Both, MHS.)

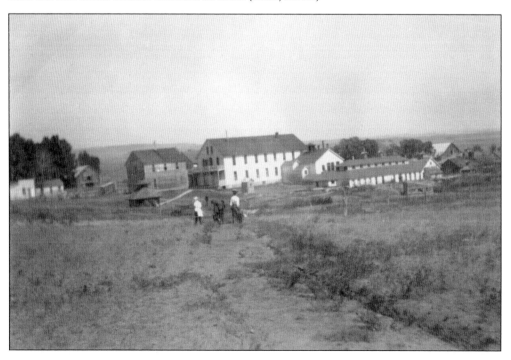

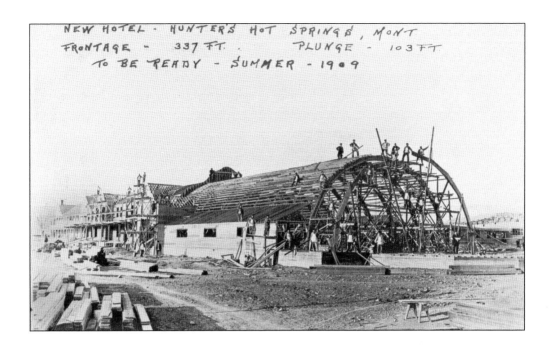

These images provide two different views of the construction of the Hotel Dakota in 1909. The old Hunter's Hot Springs Hotel was used for administrative offices after the completion of the new resort. (Both, MHS.)

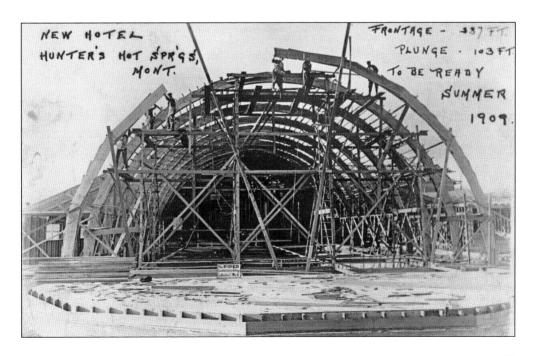

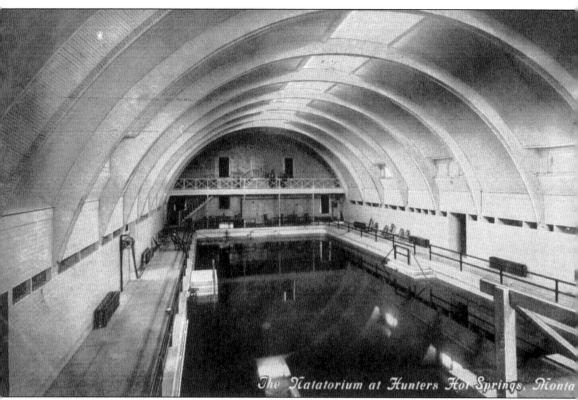

The Natatorium at Hunters Hot Springs, Montana

A "bathing department" established within the plunge building east of the hotel was complete with a sunroom, vapor baths, and private plunges. A high arched roof covered the 103-by-50-foot swimming pool, which was known as the natatorium. The pool was kept at a comfortable 85 degrees Fahrenheit. (MHS.)

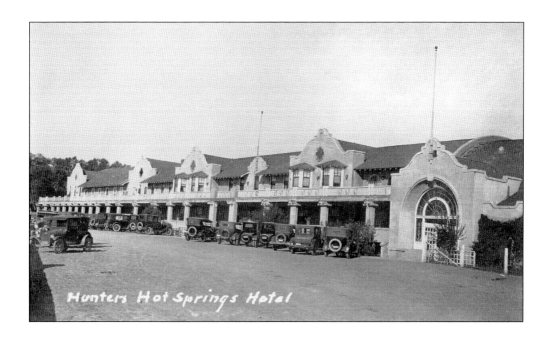

James A. Murray built the massive Hotel Dakota at Hunter's Hot Springs in 1909. Featuring five wings that could accommodate over 300 guests, the Moorish-style hotel was covered in stucco and had a two-story veranda (pictured above) that stretched for more than 400 feet. The hotel was destroyed by fire in November 1932. The attached natatorium remained open for public swimming until the early 1970s. (Both, MHS.)

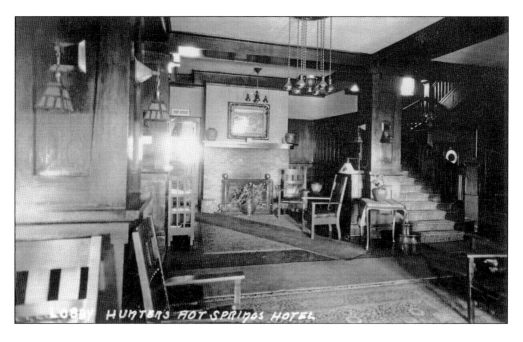

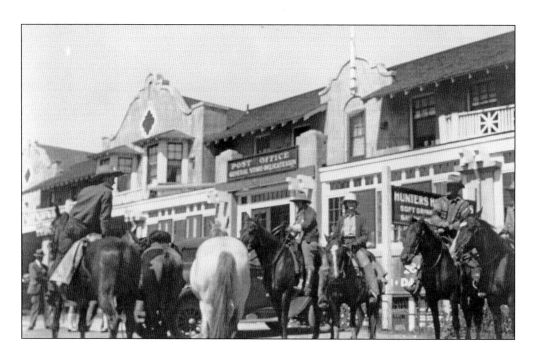

A post office occupied part of Hotel Dakota. In the early 1900s, locals would ride their horses to the resort to pick up their mail, as shown above. The Hotel Dakota was built adjacent to the stagecoach road to Yellowstone National Park. A large portion of the resort's revenue came from guests who would stay there for a day or two on their way to Yellowstone. A Northern Pacific train stopped at least four times per day at the depot about a mile south of Hunter's resort. Resort personnel would send a stage or car to take guests to and from the train station. As motorcars became more popular, visitors would often drive their own vehicles to Hunter's, where they would park next to the hotel as shown in the below photograph.

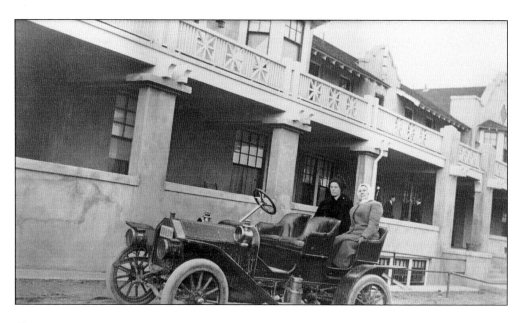

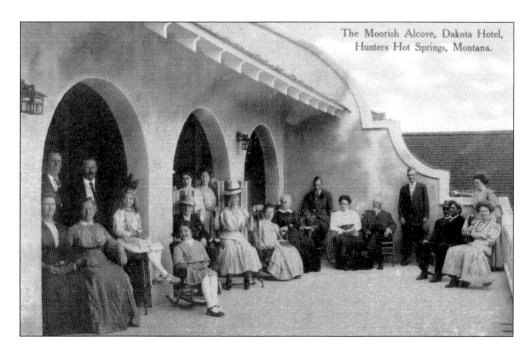

The Moorish Alcove, Dakota Hotel, Hunters Hot Springs, Montana.

Guests at the Hotel Dakota found ways to enjoy Montana's plentiful sunshine even on chilly spring and fall days. The Moorish alcove (above) occupied the end of an open-air porch on the second floor of the hotel. The south-facing alcove was sheltered from the winds, and the plentiful sunshine available in this recessed hideaway made it a popular venue for guests. At the east end of the natatorium was a light-filled solarium (below) complete with tropical ferns and potted palm trees. Bathers could relax in the solarium after using the resort's pool and soak up the sunshine that streamed through the large glass windows in the roof and south-facing wall.

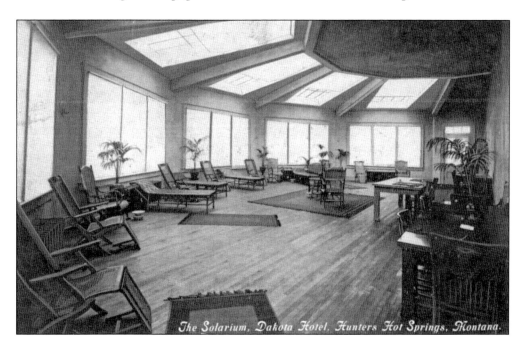

The Solarium, Dakota Hotel, Hunters Hot Springs, Montana.

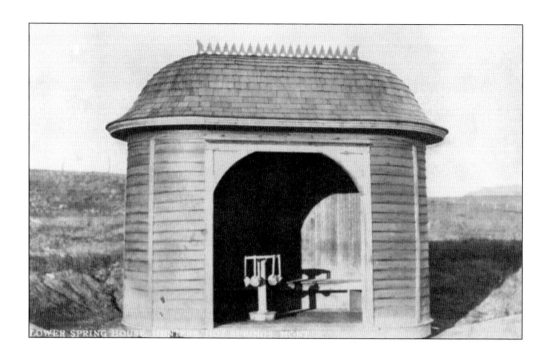

LOWER SPRING HOUSE, HUNTER'S HOT SPRINGS, MONT.

Wooden gazebos were built next to several of the artesian hot springs on the walking trails south of the hotel at Hunter's Hot Springs. In the center of each gazebo was a podium from which drinking ladles (long-handled dipping cups) were hung. Hotel guests could take a ladle and dip it into the hot springs in front of the gazebo, then drink the hot water from the filled ladle. (Both, MHS.)

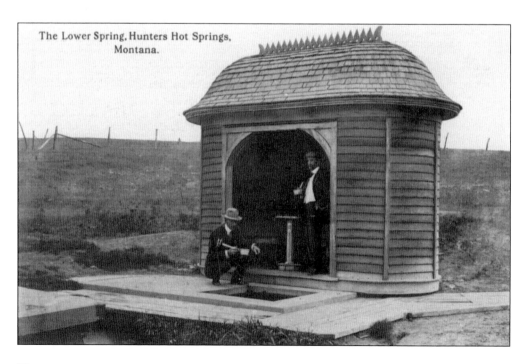

The Lower Spring, Hunters Hot Springs, Montana.

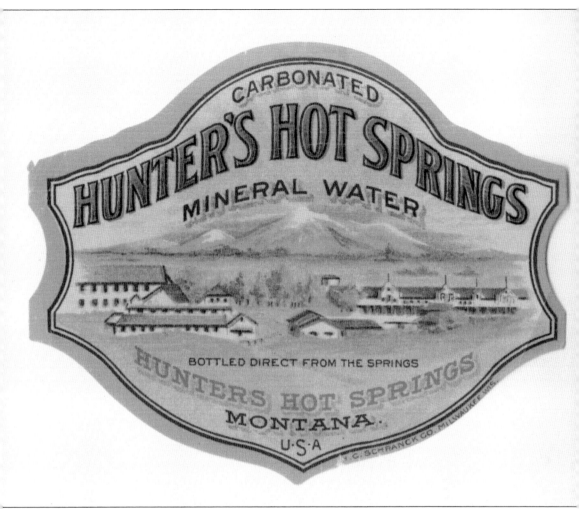

A water-bottling plant built south of the Hotel Dakota served as a base where the natural hot mineral water of Hunter's Hot Springs was bottled, labeled, and shipped across the region. Both unflavored and lemon-flavored versions of the carbonated water were bottled and sold.

The Tennis Courts at Hunters Hot Springs Hotel, Montana.

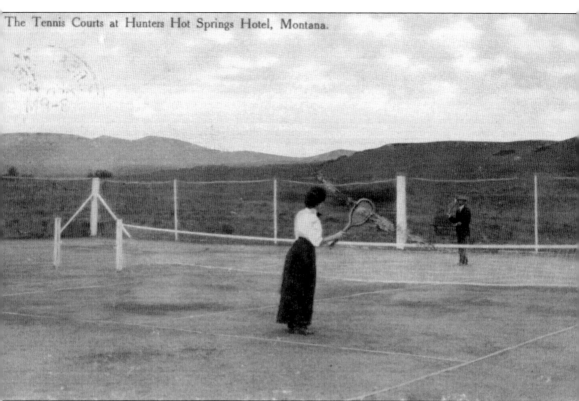

Hunter's Hot Springs was a major cultural center in Montana during the early 20th century. The Montana State Republican and Democratic conventions were held at the resort. The Montana Tennis Association gathered at Hunter's in 1909 for its annual meeting and the state tennis tournament. The tennis courts were fashioned from of a mixture of sand and molasses that hardened under the prairie sun to provide a "firm resilient surface that is unexcelled." Several state golf tournaments were also held at the resort. (MHS.)

A Corner of the Dairy, Dakota Hotel, Hunters Hot Springs, Montana.

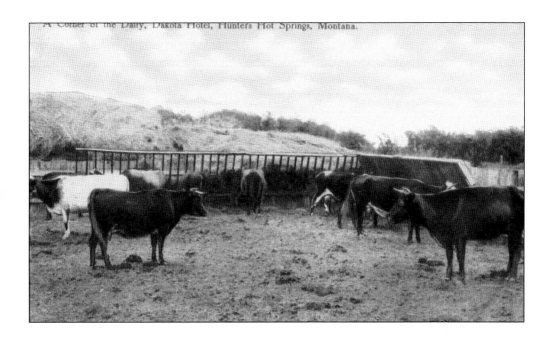

Hunter's Hot Springs had both a farm and a ranch in the early 1900s. A herd of dairy cattle kept the resort supplied with milk and cream, and locally grown beef, pork, and mutton were served at the dinner table. During the summer months, a garden supplied fresh vegetables, and a flock of hens ensured fresh eggs and fried chicken. The dining room in the Hotel Dakota contained high arched ceilings in natural fir that was stained dark green. The Mission Revival–style furniture was also stained green. The walls of the dining room were painted a deep maroon. Musicians serenaded the diners from an orchestra stage in the back of the dining room. (Above, MHS.)

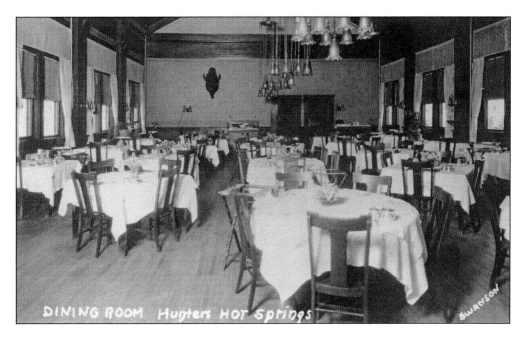

DINING ROOM Hunters HOT Springs

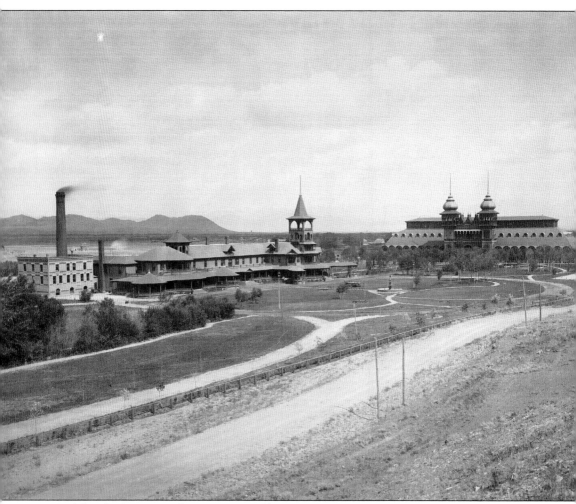

Built by Charles A. Broadwater at a cost of $500,000, the Broadwater Hotel and Natatorium, which opened in 1889, was by far Montana's most elegant spa resort. The population of the nearby town of Helena was fewer than 14,000 when the resort opened, but Broadwater thought the small town was destined to become a major city rivaling Seattle and San Francisco, which would support the sumptuous hotel and plunge. (MHS.)

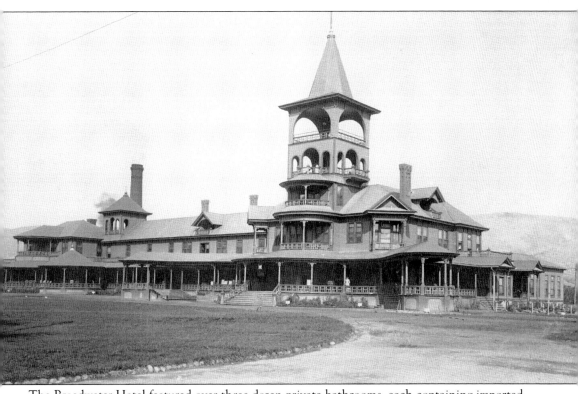

The Broadwater Hotel featured over three dozen private bathrooms, each containing imported marble therapy tubs trimmed with silver. Other health treatments offered in the hotel included spray showers called "needle baths." A guest would enter the needle bath shower, which was surrounded by metal tubes, and pinpoint streams of hot water from the tubes would then pelt the guest's body. (MHS.)

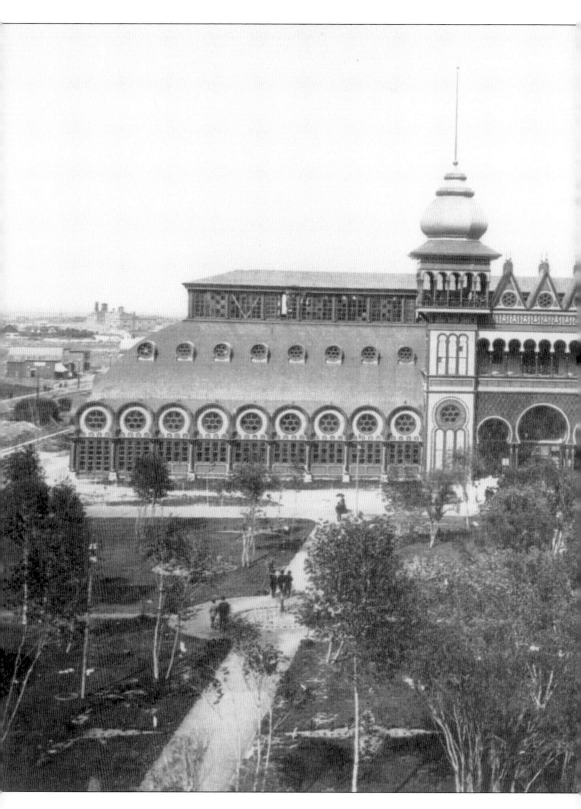

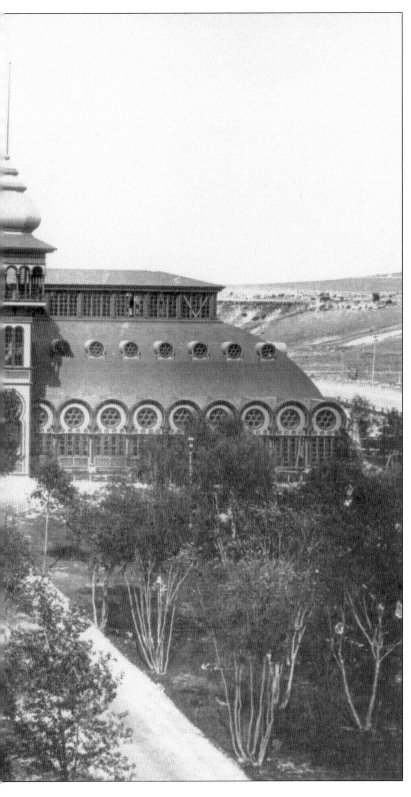

The Broadwater Natatorium, which contained a natural hot-water swimming pool larger than a football field, featured more than 12,000 square feet of windows, half of which were stained glass. The natatorium was once called the largest swimming pool in the world. The 40 acres of land surrounding the hotel and natatorium had well-manicured lawns and dozens of imported trees. More than 5,000 people attended the opening ceremonies of the resort on August 26, 1889. (MHS.)

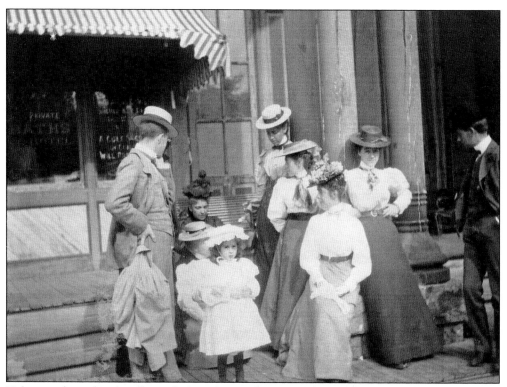

Helenians dressed in their finest clothing for social events at the Broadwater Hotel and Natatorium in the 1890s. The elegant dining room in the hotel was often turned into a ballroom where guests would enter in a grand march before dancing to local orchestras. Elaborate multicourse meals were served during special events. According to an August 27, 1889, article in the *Daily Herald*, the dining room tables were "arrayed in spotless damask and glittering with the display of silver and crystal." The menu for the dinner served during the grand opening of the hotel included lamb curry, boiled salmon, chilled oysters, prime rib, and a variety of desserts and wines. (Both, MHS.)

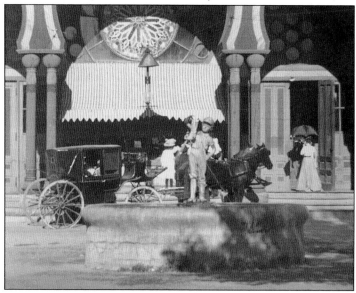

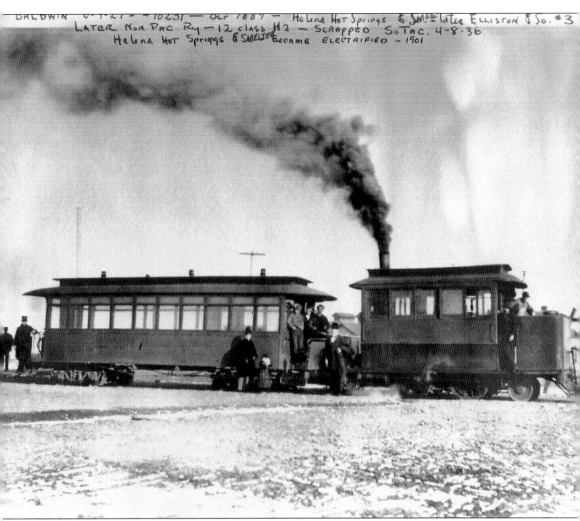

The Broadwater Hotel and Natatorium was located about 10 miles from downtown Helena—a significant journey in the 1890s. Visitors sometimes arrived by horse and buggy, but the convenience of travelling by trolley from the city center to the hot springs resort was preferred. The Helena Hot Springs and Smelter Railway started operating in 1889, the same year that the resort opened. The initial railcars were steam-powered (as shown in this photograph), but these were replaced by 1891 with cleaner electric-powered trolleys. The trolleys could make the trip from downtown Helena to the hot springs in about 20 minutes. (MHS.)

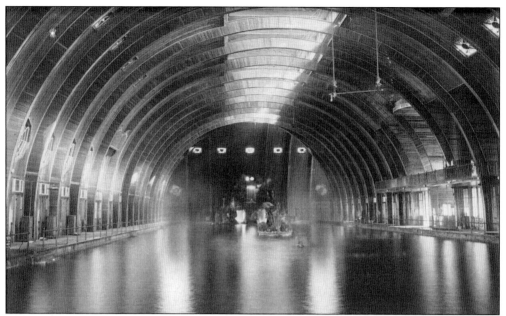

These photographs show the interior of the Broadwater Natatorium. During the opening weekend of the resort in 1889, the *Helena Weekly Herald* reported that "the great plunge was crowded with bathers, and at all times presented the appearance of a pool covered with heavy raindrops, so thickly was it studded with heads." (Both, MHS.)

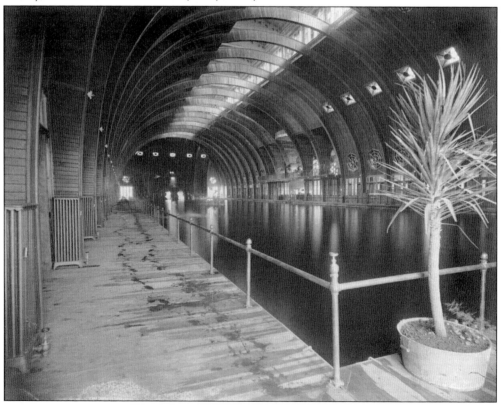

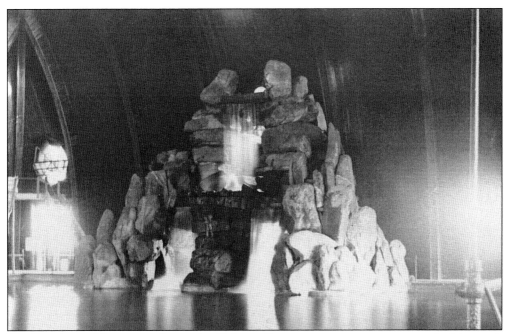

The Broadwater Natatorium featured a 40-foot-tall granite outcropping at one end of the pool. Twin waterfalls cascaded from the sides of the outcropping—one waterfall of cold water and one of hot water. Sealed electric lamps lit the waterfalls from behind. Adventurous guests could climb to the top of the outcropping and dive into the deep pool below. (MHS.)

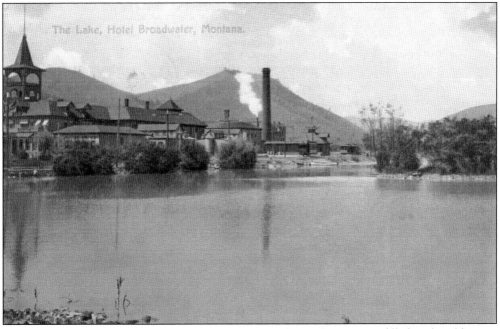

Lake Thermal, a 12-foot-deep pond behind the Hotel Broadwater, was filled with cold water from nearby Ten-Mile Creek. Lake Thermal was also called Lake Wilder, named after Charles Broadwater's daughter. Hotel guests could paddle canoes and rowboats around the lake before retiring to the hotel for dinner and a good night's sleep. (MHS.)

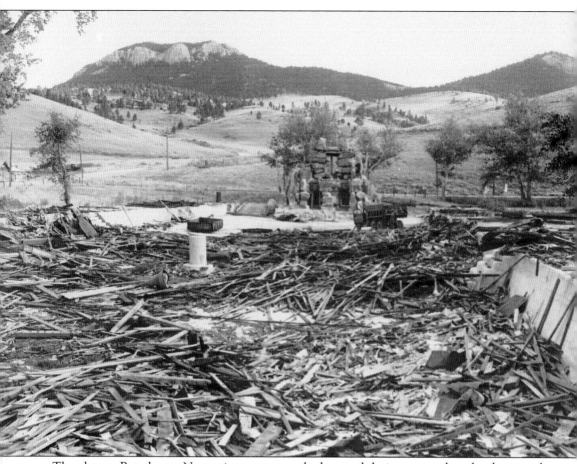

The elegant Broadwater Natatorium was severely damaged during an earthquake that struck Helena in 1935, and the structure was demolished soon thereafter. In this photograph, a dump truck is dwarfed by the ruins of the 40-foot-tall granite waterfall that once filled the swimming pool with a mixture of cold and hot water. Mount Helena rises in the background. (MHS.)

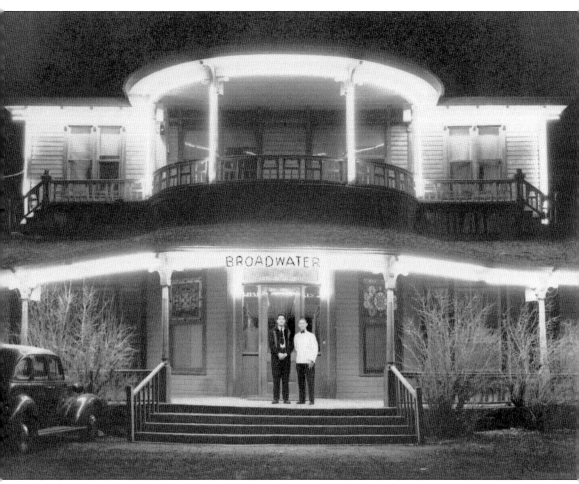

The Broadwater Hotel suffered financial losses almost from the date of its grand opening in the summer of 1889. The resort's founder, Charles A. Broadwater, died only three years after the grand opening, and the resort languished without his guidance and vision. The Broadwater Hotel shut its doors in 1895 after being in operation for fewer than 10 years, but it was briefly reopened as a nightclub in the 1930s until it was again closed during Prohibition. The hotel then sat empty for almost 40 years until it was demolished in the 1970s. (MHS.)

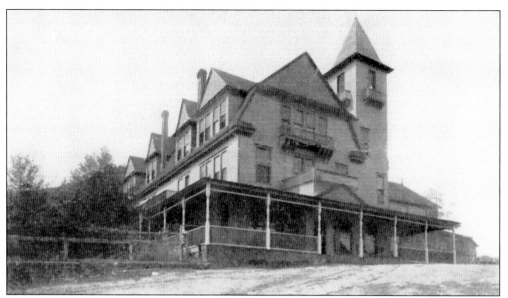

Prospector James Riley claimed Boulder Hot Springs in 1863. A small hotel was built near the springs by 1881. C.W. Kerrick secured a 10-year lease on the property in 1891 and built the three-story hotel pictured above. The building, named the Hotel May, contained 52 guest rooms, a billiards room, and an amusement hall. (MHS.)

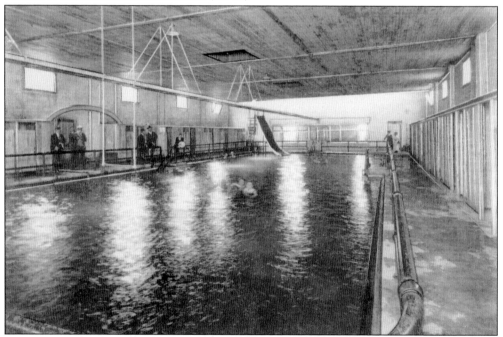

The Boulder Hot Springs plunge is pictured here around 1890. The *Butte Miner* reported that "The plunge is filled with the health-giving fluid of the most ravishing temperature, into which the pleasure-seekers, regardless of sex, plunge and swim and float around in a heterogeneous mass and in perfect ecstasy." A local newspaper reported at the time that soaking in the hot water at Boulder Hot Springs was an "absolute cure for rheumatism, dyspepsia, and all disease of the digestive organs." (MHS.)

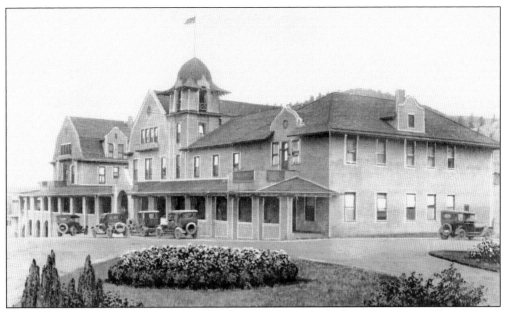

Moorish-style architecture was common at hot springs resorts built in the western United States in the late 19th and early 20th centuries. James A. Murray expanded the Hotel May in 1919, including Moorish themes in the exterior design as well as Arts and Crafts interiors. The expanded building was renamed the Boulder Hot Springs Hotel. In the 1920s and 1930s, the Boulder Hot Springs Hotel featured immaculate landscaping that added to the perception of elegance about the resort. (MHS.)

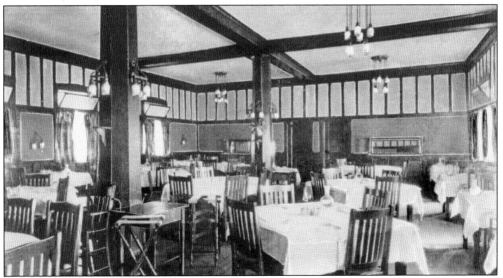

The dining room in the Boulder Hot Springs Hotel is pictured here around 1910. The dining room featured ornate decorations, including amber lampshades made by Tiffany & Co. and wall stencils in an Arts and Crafts design. Mission Revival–style oak tables and chairs filled the dining area. The adjacent 40-by-80-foot front lobby was also decorated in the Arts and Crafts style, with comfortable couches for lounging after dinner. The *Helena Record* noted the popularity of the restaurant in the 1920s, reporting on "the number of Butte cars, among the scores from all over Hades and half of Texas, parked around the place on a Sunday afternoon." (MHS.)

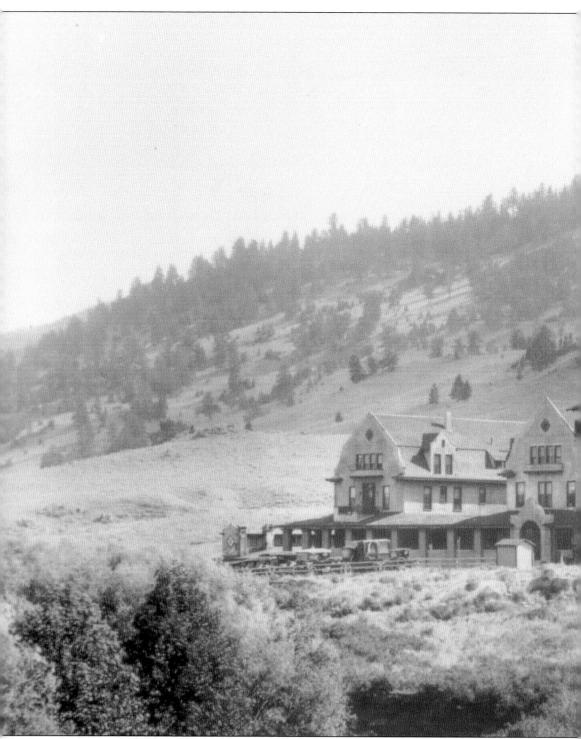

Butte millionaire James Murray purchased the Boulder Hot Springs Hotel from C.W. Kerrick in 1909, expanding the structure with new guest wings as well as a bar and ballroom. "Pappy" Smith purchased the hotel from Murray in 1940, renaming it the "Diamond S Ranchotel," which he

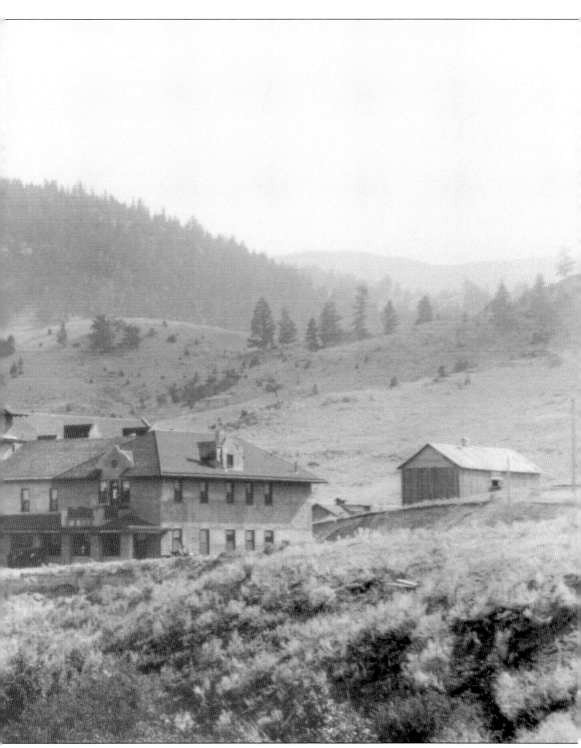

managed until 1960. The hotel fell into disrepair in the 1970s and 1980s but was renovated and turned into a retreat and teaching center in the 1990s. (MHS.)

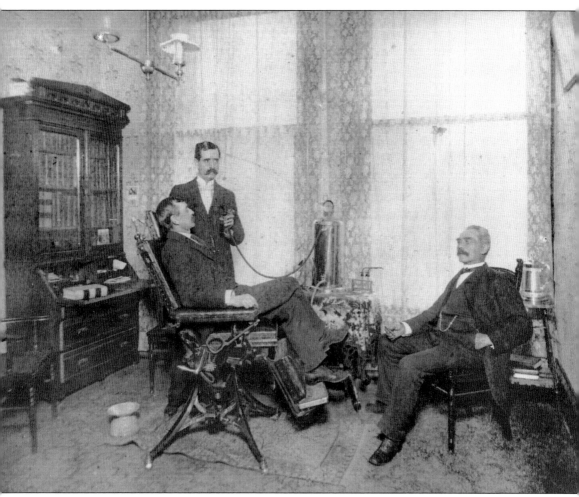

A variety of medical treatments were offered at Boulder Hot Springs in the 1890s, including a procedure called the "Keeley Cure." Dr. Leslie Keeley, of Illinois, convinced his patients that he could quickly cure them of addictions to "liquor, opium, morphine, chloral, cocaine, cigarette and tobacco habits." Keeley's unorthodox approach included injecting bichloride of gold into a patient's arm four times a day. Dr. Keeley boasted that his treatment for alcoholism was so effective that "if a new arrival needs whiskey, it is given to him in a bottle, and he can have more until his palate loathes it and he returns his unopened bottle to the doctor." (MHS.)

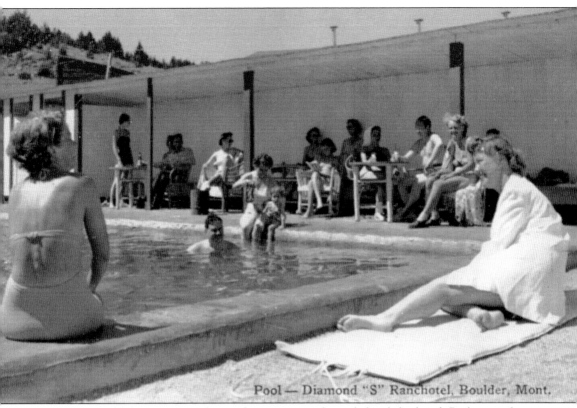

Pool — Diamond "S" Ranchotel, Boulder, Mont.

After 1940, Boulder Hot Springs featured an open-air plunge behind the hotel. Bathers at the renamed Diamond S Ranchotel could take advantage of massages, dancing, dining, fishing, and hiking. A Sunday night smorgasbord was a regular attraction for hotel guests during the 1960s. (MHS.)

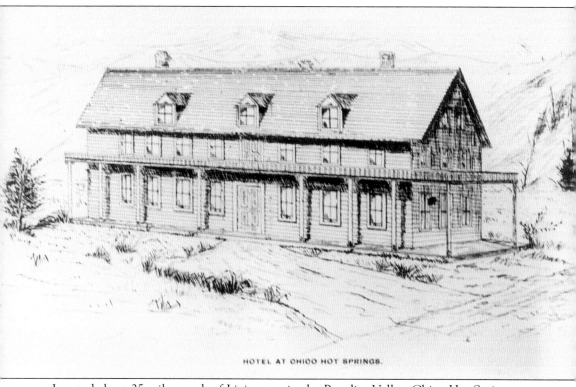

HOTEL AT CHICO HOT SPRINGS.

Located about 25 miles south of Livingston in the Paradise Valley, Chico Hot Springs was a local secret until the late 1880s. William Knowles purchased the springs in 1899 and opened the first hotel in June 1900. This image shows a line drawing of the first hotel plan for Chico Hot Springs. (YGM.)

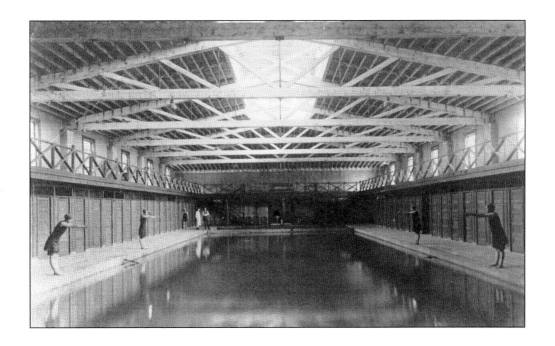

William Knowles built a covered swimming pool behind the Chico Hot Springs Hotel in 1919. The ceiling of the pool was vented to allow moisture to escape. The image below shows a concrete divider between pool sections. The smaller pool in the foreground was filled with hot water in which guests could soak away their aches and pains. The larger pool was cooled for swimming. Dressing rooms were located at the back of the pool. (Above, MHS; below, YGM.)

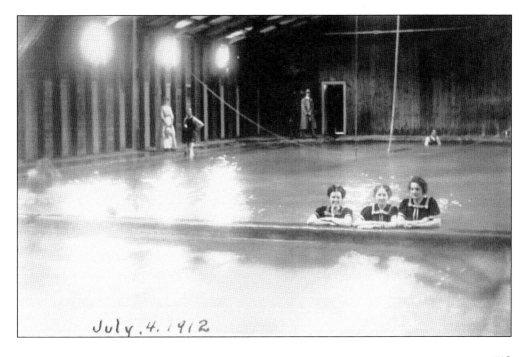

July. 4. 1912

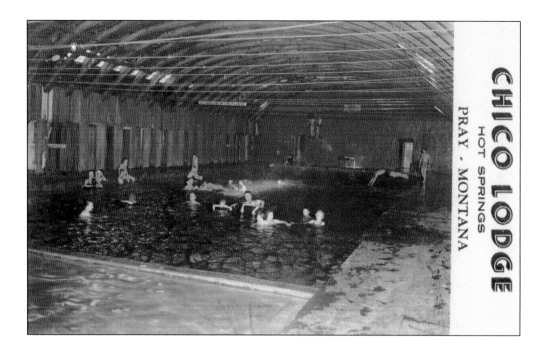

Above is another picture of the covered pool built at Chico Hot Springs in 1919. The aerial view of the Chico Hot Springs resort on the below postcard shows the covered pool attached to the back of the lodge. The pool roof collapsed in 1957. (Both, MHS.)

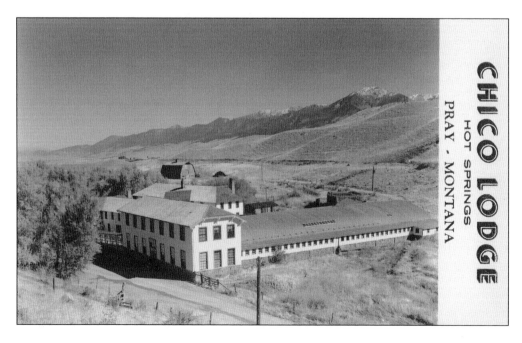

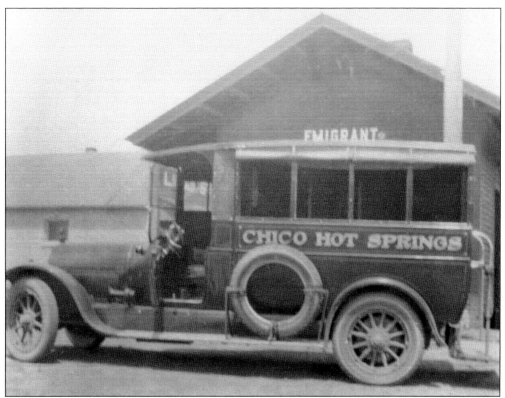

Guests arriving by rail were met at the train station in Emigrant about four miles from the resort. The above image shows a Cadillac automobile that the Chico resort used for a shuttle around 1917. Many guests arrived at Chico Hot Springs in their own automobiles, even in the early 1900s, as shown in the below photograph. (Both, YGM.)

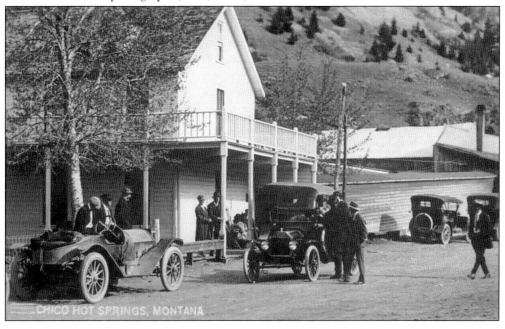

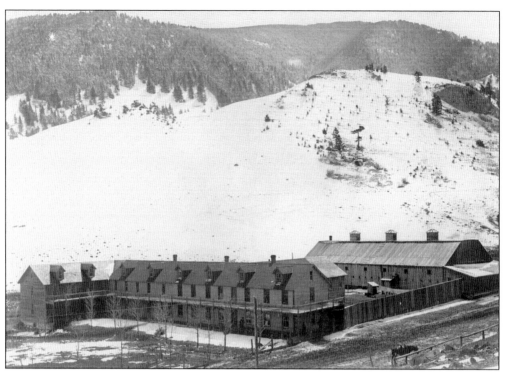

During the winter of 1914–1915, a two-dormer wing was added to the back of the Chico Hot Springs Hotel. The new rooms served as offices and examining rooms for Dr. G.A. Townsend, the resort's resident physician from 1912 to 1925. The resort's former physician, Dr. F.E. Corwin, practiced at Chico from 1900 until 1908. Corwin left Chico to develop his own hot springs resort, which he named Corwin Hot Springs Hotel (see pages 120–126). (YGM.)

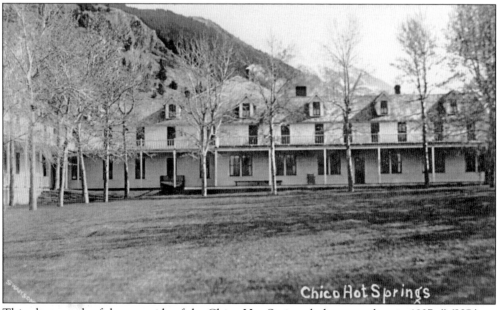

This photograph of the west side of the Chico Hot Springs lodge was taken in 1927. (MHS.)

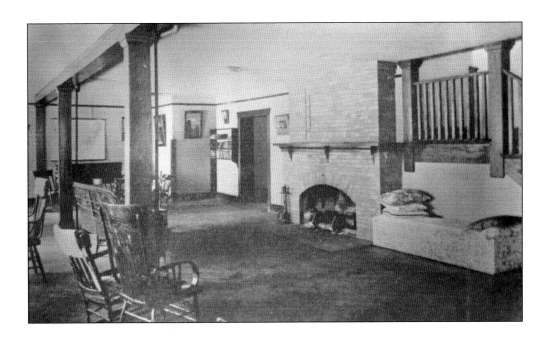

These images present two views of the lobby at the Chico Hot Springs Hotel. The above photograph shows the lobby around 1920, and the below image shows the lobby in the 1940s. The lobby bustled with the energy of arriving and departing guests and was the gateway to the popular Chico dining room. The stairs on the far left led up to the guest rooms. (Both, MHS.)

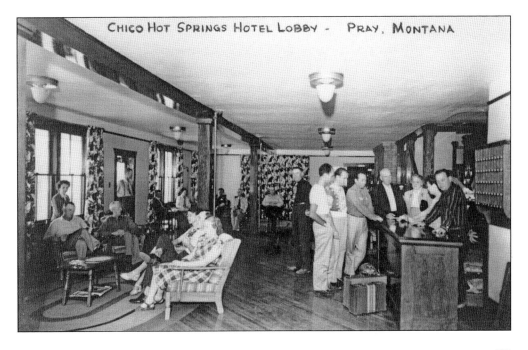

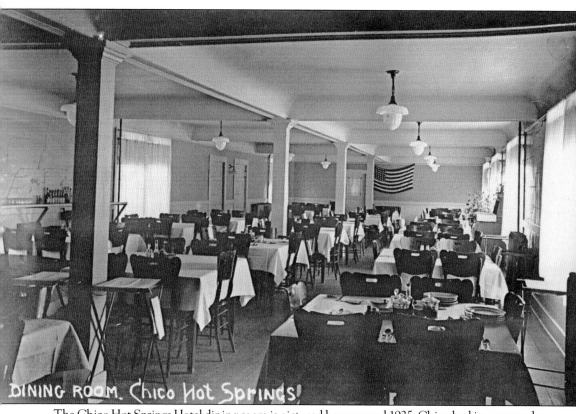

DINING ROOM. Chico Hot Springs!

The Chico Hot Springs Hotel dining room is pictured here around 1925. Chico had its own garden and a dairy herd and supplied much of the food served in the hotel dining room. The restaurant developed a reputation for offering one of the best dining experiences in Montana.

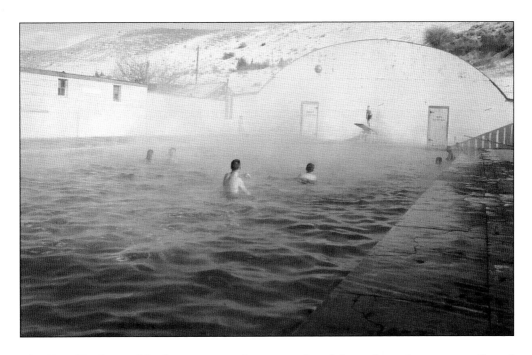

The Chico Hot Springs Hotel swimming pool was covered until the roof over the structure collapsed on May 30, 1957. Instead of replacing the roof, Chico's owners decided to leave the pool open to the sky. These two photographs from the 1960s show the open-air pool from both ends.

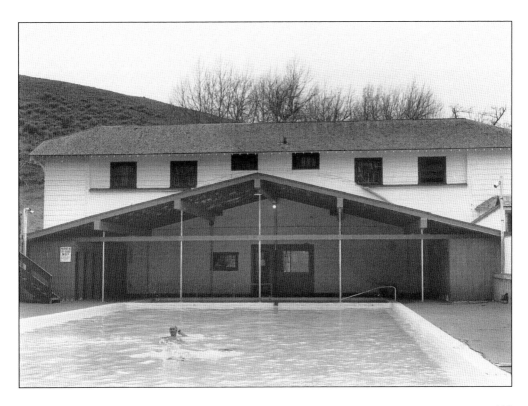

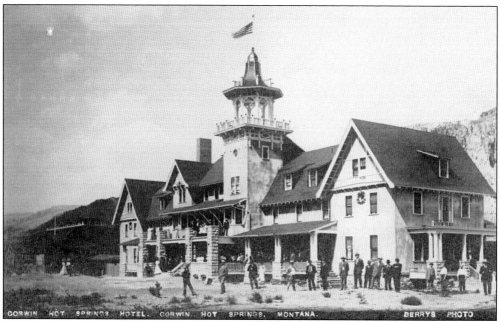

The Corwin Hot Springs Hotel is shown in these two images. The hotel was built in 1909. Physician F.E. Corwin purchased the LaDuke Hot Springs from Julius LaDuke in 1908 (see page 11). Dr. Corwin opened the Corwin Hot Springs Hotel and Sanitarium in 1909. Located nine miles north of Yellowstone National Park, the 86-room hotel had many design elements similar to resorts Dr. Corwin had seen during visits he had taken to Austria. The hotel featured electric lights and telephones in each room—a rarity in the 1900s in Montana. Electricity for the resort was provided by a hydropower generator in a stream located a few miles away in the mountains surrounding the resort. At night, the hotel twinkled with electric lights, which led the *Livingston Enterprise* to report that "tourists passing by would think they had passed through fairyland." (Above, MHS.)

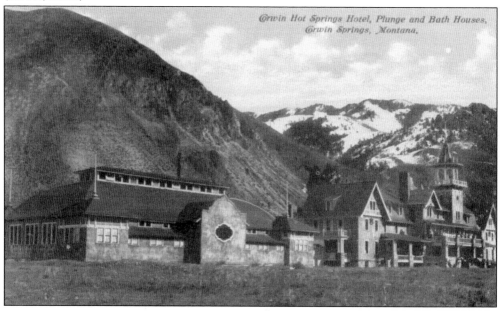

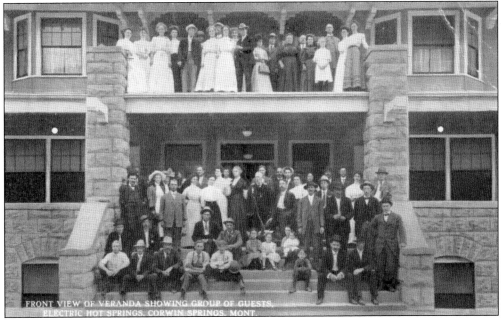

This photograph of the veranda and entrance to the Corwin Hot Springs Hotel was taken in 1909. Guests are gathered on both the upper and lower stories of the hotel. (MHS.)

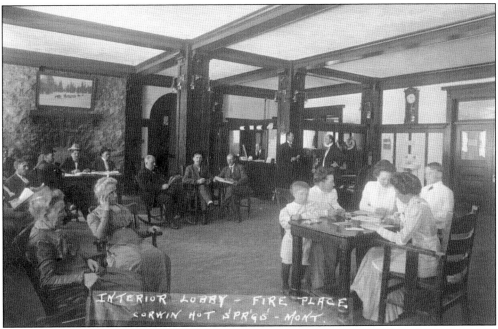

The interior lobby of the Corwin Hot Springs Hotel provided a gathering place for visitors. Men enjoyed reading the newspaper near the hotel fireplace, while women engaged in conversation and letter-writing at nearby tables. New arrivals could be observed checking in at the reception area. Like many resorts in the early 1900s, the Corwin Hotel lobby featured furniture and construction in the popular Arts and Crafts style. (MHS.)

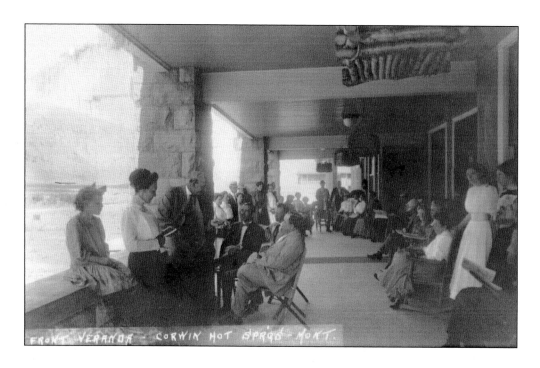

On a warm summer day, hotel guests would socialize on the Corwin Hotel veranda, engaging in conversation while sitting in rocking chairs or on the low veranda wall. When the resort opened in 1909, visitors gathered in large numbers from the nearby town of Gardiner. However, the hotel had difficulty attracting a consistently large crowd, and within a year of its opening, it began to lose money. A bank in Livingston eventually foreclosed on the property. (Both, MHS.)

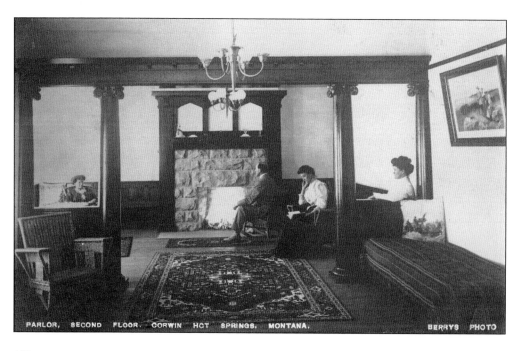

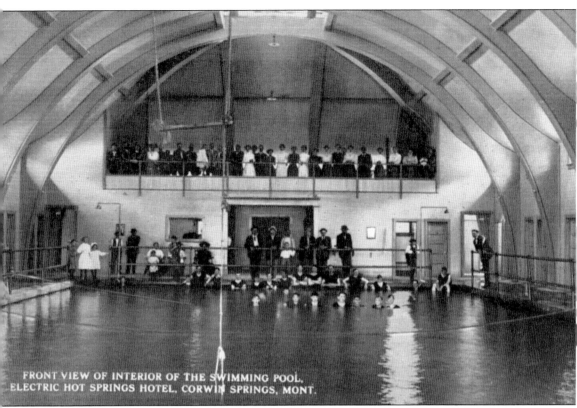

FRONT VIEW OF INTERIOR OF THE SWIMMING POOL,
ELECTRIC HOT SPRINGS HOTEL, CORWIN SPRINGS, MONT.

A 50-by-80-foot enclosed swimming pool was built adjacent to the Corwin Hot Springs Hotel. Hot water was transported to the pool through wooden pipes from LaDuke Hot Springs, located two miles upstream on the banks of the Yellowstone River. The hot water was continuously piped through the bathing pool, providing a complete change of water every six minutes. Vapor baths, plunge baths, and private soaking rooms were also available. Visitors in the early 1900s paid about $15 per week for room and board in the hotel and to partake in hot-water soaks. (MHS.)

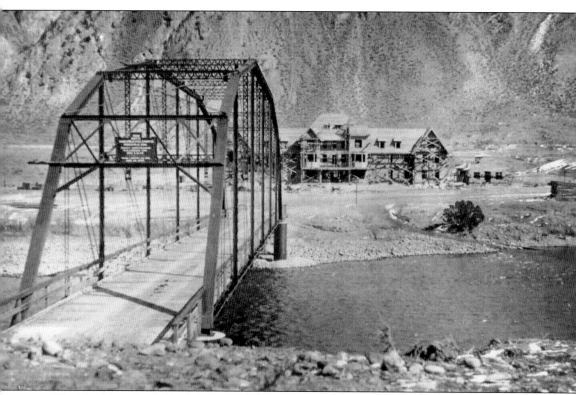

The Northern Pacific Railway made daily stops to drop off passengers on the opposite side of the Yellowstone River from the Corwin Hot Springs Hotel. Owner Dr. F.E. Corwin partnered with Park County to build an iron bridge—at a cost of $13,500—that would transport passengers from the rail stop across the Yellowstone River to the resort. One of the advertised attractions of the hotel was the fire-protection system, which consisted of hydrants installed at the four corners of the hotel, "from any of which a stream can be thrown over the top of the structure," according to the *Livingston Post*. In spite of the vaunted fire-protection system, the Corwin Hot Springs Hotel burned to the ground in 1916, only seven years after it opened. The resort was valued at $100,000 before the fire, but the owners only carried $50,000 in fire insurance and were unable to rebuild. (YGM.)

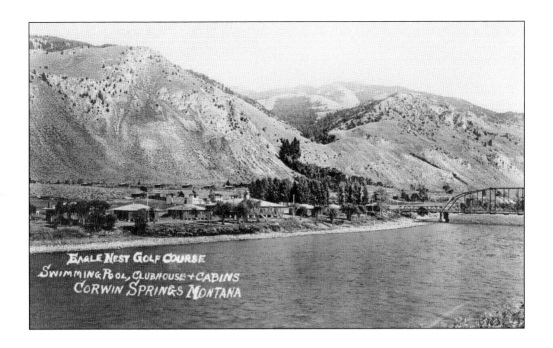

Following the devastating fire that destroyed the original resort in 1916, Walter J. Hill of the Northern Pacific Railway purchased the Corwin Hot Springs property in 1920. Construction of a new resort followed, and in April 1922, Hill held the grand opening of the Eagle's Nest Dude Ranch. The Western-themed resort featured a clubhouse, a nine-hole golf course, a restaurant, a dance hall, and an open-air plunge. (Both, MHS.)

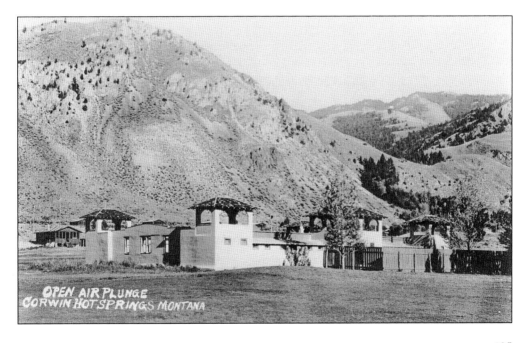

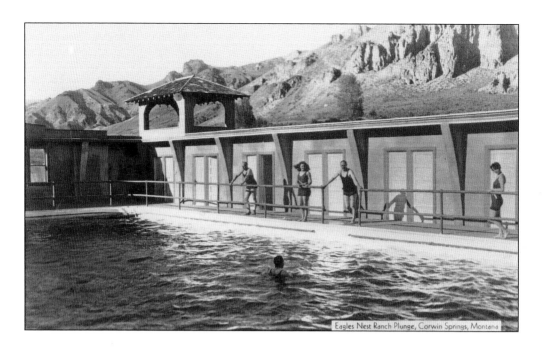

Eagles Nest Ranch Plunge, Corwin Springs, Montana

The Mission Revival–style open-air plunge at the Eagle's Nest Dude Ranch was filled with hot water piped from the LaDuke Hot Springs in the same way that the old Corwin Hot Springs resort had used the water. The 70-by-115-foot plunge for the dude ranch opened in 1922. The resort closed in the 1940s. After the resort closed, the hot springs and property remained unused until the 1980s, when a religious group called the Church Universal and Triumphant purchased the property and incorporated it into their headquarters for the Royal Teton Ranch. (Above, MHS; below, YGM.)

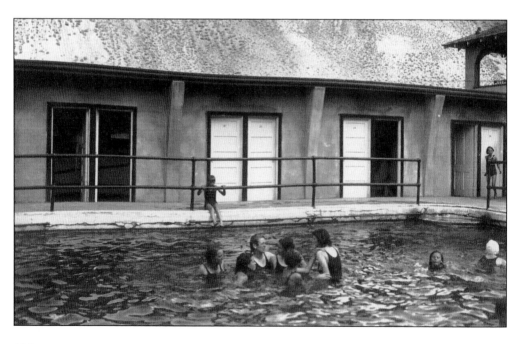

INDEX

DISCOVER THOUSANDS OF LOCAL HISTORY BOOKS
FEATURING MILLIONS OF VINTAGE IMAGES

Arcadia Publishing, the leading local history publisher in the United States, is committed to making history accessible and meaningful through publishing books that celebrate and preserve the heritage of America's people and places.

Find more books like this at
www.arcadiapublishing.com

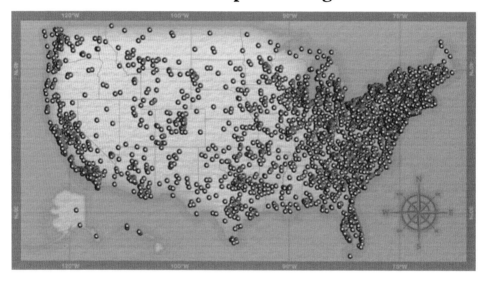

Search for your hometown history, your old stomping grounds, and even your favorite sports team.

Consistent with our mission to preserve history on a local level, this book was printed in South Carolina on American-made paper and manufactured entirely in the United States. Products carrying the accredited Forest Stewardship Council (FSC) label are printed on 100 percent FSC-certified paper.

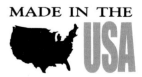

MADE IN THE USA